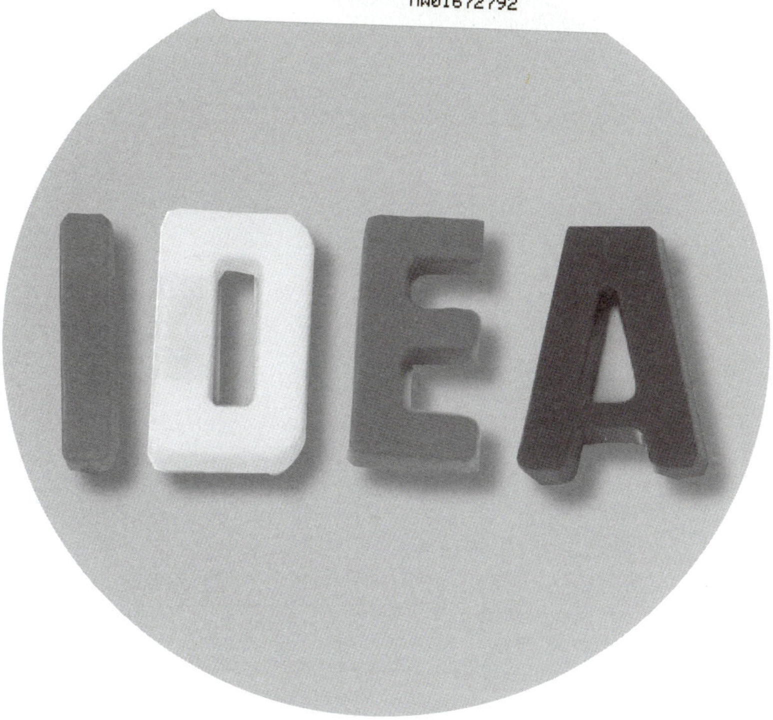

Providing Physical Therapy Services

Under Parts B & C of the Individuals With Disabilities Education Act (IDEA)

Irene R McEwen, PT, PhD, FAPTA, Editor

University of Oklahoma Health Sciences Center, Department of Rehabilitation Sciences:
Irene R McEwen, PT, PhD, FAPTA, Editor
Sandra Arnold, PT, PhD
Elizabeth DeGrace, PhD, OTR/L
Lynn Jeffries, PT, PhD, PCS
Maria Jones, PT, PhD, ATP
Thubi H A Kolobe, PT, PhD
Amanda Porter, PT, MPT
Julie D Smith, MS, OTR/L
Lorraine Sylvester, PT, MS

University of Colorado Department of Physical Medicine and Rehabilitation:
Mary Jane Rapport, PT, PhD

University of Central Oklahoma:
Traci Castles

Accompanying this copy of ***Providing Physical Therapy Services Under Parts B & C of the Individuals With Disabilities Education Act (IDEA)*** is a CD with the contents of Assistance to States for the Education of Children With Disabilities and Preschool Grants for Children With Disabilities; *Federal Register 34 CFR Part 300* (Final Rule, August 14, 2006) and *34 CFR Part 303* (Proposed Rule, May 9, 2007).

CD INSTRUCTIONS The document on the accompanying CD is a PDF file and requires Adobe Reader. If Adobe Reader is already installed, follow the instructions below for Windows or Macintosh platforms. To install or upgrade to the latest version of Adobe Reader, go to http://www.adobe.com/products/reader and download the free software.

WINDOWS Insert the CD-ROM into your CD/DVD drive. The disk will AutoRun and prompt you at the Main Menu. If there is no prompt, open My Computer and double-click to open the removable drive that contains the CD, then follow the prompts on the main menu.

MACINTOSH Insert the CD-ROM into your CD/DVD drive, open the OSX folder and double-click on the Start.pdf file to begin, or, when the icon for the CD appears on the screen, double-click to open, then click on the Start.pdf file.

ISBN 978-0-9702105-1-7

www.pediatricapta.org

Table of Contents

Second Edition Preface and Acknowledgments

This book is the fourth in a series of documents that the Section on Pediatrics of the American Physical Therapy Association (APTA) has published over the past 27 years about provision of physical therapy under the Individuals With Disabilities Education Act and prior related legislation. The preface to the first edition of this book describes the previous documents and their chronology.

This second edition provides an update and expansion of the first edition, with much of the new content in response to questions we have received from readers of the first edition. Major changes include: (1) updates related to the Individuals With Disabilities Education Improvement Act Amendments of 2004 and its regulations; (2) new chapters on parent-professional collaboration, early intervention in natural environments, and transportation; and (3) contributions by several new authors.

Important Note: At the time this book went to press in January 2009, the final regulations for Part C of the Individuals With Disabilities Education Improvement Act of 2004 were not yet available. To avoid delaying publication any longer while waiting for the final regulations, we decided to proceed using the *proposed* Part C regulations. Although we do not anticipate major changes in the regulations cited in this book, the final regulations may differ somewhat from the proposed regulations. For this reason, readers should check the final regulations when they become available. The US Department of Education Web site at **http://idea.ed.gov** is a good source of information about the regulations and other aspects of IDEA. You may also check the APTA Web site at **www.apta.org/idea**. After the final regulations become available, we will review them for any differences in the regulations cited in this book and post the information on the Section on Pediatrics Web site at **www.pediatricapta.org**.

CONTRIBUTORS

Sandra Arnold, PT, PhD

Sandra Arnold is clinical assistant professor in the Department of Rehabilitation Sciences at the University of Oklahoma Health Sciences Center and formerly served as the director of occupational therapy and physical therapy programs for the Oklahoma State Department of Education for 12 years. In addition to teaching in the professional programs in physical therapy and occupational therapy and the post-professional program in rehabilitation sciences, she provides continuing education locally and nationally in the area of school-based related services. Arnold also serves on the editorial board of *Physical & Occupational Therapy in Pediatrics*.

Traci Castles, BS
Traci Castles is the mother of 3 children who have disabilities. She is the cofounder of Oklahoma's parent-to-parent program, Oklahoma Family Network, and a state coordinator for Family Voices in Oklahoma. Castles served 5 ½ years as family faculty for the Tolbert Center for Developmental Disabilities, Department of Rehabilitation Sciences, University of Oklahoma Health Sciences Center. During that time she provided a family perspective in professional and postprofessional coursework, participated in development of the STARS training program, and served as an agency coordinator for SoonerStart, Oklahoma's early intervention program. Currently, Castles is a public relations director and a licensed marriage and family therapy (LMFT) candidate at the University of Central Oklahoma.

Elizabeth DeGrace, PhD, OTR/L
Elizabeth DeGrace is assistant professor in the Department of Rehabilitation Sciences at the University of Oklahoma Health Sciences Center. She teaches in the professional occupational therapy and physical therapy programs and the postprofessional programs in rehabilitation sciences. Most of her teaching relates to children with disabilities and their families, and her research focuses on family experiences following a diagnosis of autism. She also provides technical assistance for SoonerStart, Oklahoma's early intervention program, for families who have children with autism.

Lynn Jeffries, PT, PhD, PCS
Lynn Jeffries is clinical assistant professor in the Department of Rehabilitation Sciences at the University of Oklahoma Health Sciences Center. In addition to teaching in the department's professional and postprofessional programs, she is the director of a program that provides training about children with disabilities for child care providers and provides state-wide consultation, services, and personnel development for SoonerStart, Oklahoma's early intervention program. She also is the Oklahoma coordinator for a multisite international research project examining the motor, self-care, and play skills of young children with cerebral palsy.

Maria Jones, PT, PhD, ATP
Maria Jones is clinical assistant professor in the Department of Rehabilitation Sciences at the University of Oklahoma Health Sciences Center. She is credentialed as an assistive technology practitioner (ATP) through the Rehabilitation Engineering and Assistive Technology Society of North America (RESNA). Her primary research interests are the use of power mobility for young children with severe motor impairments and assistive technology. Jones teaches postprofessional courses in assistive technology and has made many presentations to professional audiences. She consults with SoonerStart, Oklahoma's early intervention program, the Oklahoma State Department of Education, the Oklahoma Developmental Disabilities Services Division, and the Oklahoma Health Care in the area of assistive technology and other services for people with developmental disabilities.

Thubi H A Kolobe, PT, PhD
Thubi Kolobe is a professor in the Department of Rehabilitation Science at the University of Oklahoma Health Sciences Center. Her teaching, practice, and research interests are with children with disabilities and their families, particularly children 0–3 years of age. She has published in the areas of developmental tests, childrearing practices, and family-centered intervention. Kolobe is a co-author of the *Test of Infant Motor Performance*, a motor test for preterm and very young infants. Her current research include the impact of the caregiving environment on child development and performance, early identification of infants at risk for developmental disabilities, and self-initiated mobility in infants with cerebral palsy.

Irene McEwen, PT, PhD, FAPTA
Irene McEwen holds the Ann Taylor Chair in Pediatrics and Developmental Disabilities in Physical Therapy in the Department of Rehabilitation Sciences at the University of Oklahoma Health Sciences Center. She teaches pediatrics, evidence-based practice, and research in the department's professional occupational therapy and physical therapy education programs and the postprofessional program in rehabilitation sciences. She is

project director of a training grant from the US Department of Education that provides a fully Web-based Master of Science degree program in early intervention, school-based practice, and assistive technology for physical therapists and occupational therapists. She has published and conducted research related to school-based practice and assistive technology for children with severe disabilities.

Amanda Porter, PT, MPT
Amanda Porter is assistive technology curriculum specialist in the Department of Rehabilitation Sciences at the University of Oklahoma Health Sciences Center. She works with the department's Oklahoma Assistive Technology Center on a contract with the Oklahoma State Department of Education. The contract supports a program of training and technical assistance for teachers, support staff, and related service providers to increase their knowledge of assistive technology services for students with disabilities and assists Oklahoma public schools to meet the assistive technology requirements of IDEA. A component of the program provides assistive technology consultation and assessment in Oklahoma Public Schools.

Mary Jane Rapport, PT, PhD
Mary Jane Rapport is a professor in the School of Medicine, Department of Physical Medicine and Rehabilitation at the University of Colorado. She is the assistant director of the physical therapy program and is active in the American Physical Therapy Association (APTA) and the APTA Section on Pediatrics. Rapport has published and presented nationally on the topic of school-based practice and early intervention.

Julie D Smith, MS, OTR/L
Julie Smith is the assistant director of the Oklahoma Autism Network in the Department of Rehabilitation Sciences at the University of Oklahoma Health Sciences Center. She formerly was the program director of Statewide Training and Regional Supports, a personnel development program for professionals working with infants and toddlers, preschoolers and students ages 6 through 21 with disabilities. Smith provides training and technical assistance for development of the individualized family service plans, early childhood transition from SoonerStart to school and community services, evidence-based practice, parent-child interaction, sensory processing, and supporting children with challenging behaviors/autism and their families. She has provided early intervention and school-based services.

Lorraine Sylvester, PT, MS
Lorraine Sylvester is a physical therapist in the Department of Rehabilitation Sciences at the University of Oklahoma Health Sciences Center and a research assistant at the Zarrow Center for Learning Enrichment in the Educational Psychology Department at the University of Oklahoma, where she is pursing her doctoral degree. Her doctoral research investigates the relationship between physical therapy interventions, self-determination, and transition to postsecondary life for youth with severe and multiple disabilities.

The preface to the first edition acknowledges and thanks many people who contributed to the book. We continue to thank them and also several others. We thank M'Lisa Shelden, who was one of the authors of the first edition and contributed particularly to the chapters on transition and individualized family service plans. We also thank the board of directors of the Section on Pediatrics of the American Physical Therapy Association, who encouraged and supported publication of a second edition, and Cindy Sliwa, Section on Pediatrics executive officer, who so capably facilitated the publication process.

First Edition Preface and Acknowledgments

This book is the third in a series of documents on provision of physical therapy services in educational environments that the Section on Pediatrics of the American Physical Therapy Association (APTA) has published over the past 20 years. The first document, titled *Physical Therapy Practice in Educational Environments: Policies, Guidelines, and Background Information*, was published in 1980. Members of the Section on Pediatrics wrote the 1980 document in response to members' requests for more information about service delivery under Public Law 94-142, the Education for All Handicapped Children Act, passed by the United States Congress in 1975.

Over the years, the first document became out-of-date. The Act was amended, due process hearings and court cases clarified the law, and "best practices" in special education and related services were redefined. Between 1988 and 1990 a subcommittee of the Education Committee of the APTA Section on Pediatrics revised the original document. Karen D Martin, who was instrumental in writing the 1980 document, edited the 1990 revision, titled *Physical Therapy Practice in Educational Environments: Policies and Guidelines.*

Time passed and the 1990 document also became out-of-date. The name of the Act was changed to Individuals With Disabilities Education Act (IDEA); assistive technology and other services were added to the law; children with autism or traumatic brain injury became eligible for services; and early intervention services (now Part C, formerly Part H) were implemented across the country. Pediatric physical therapy also has changed since 1990. Practice is now more family-focused and team-oriented. Treatments now place greater emphasis on systems and motor learning approaches. Members of the APTA Section on Pediatrics again requested that the publication be updated to provide more current information.

At first we attempted to revise the 1990 document using the same format. We soon discovered, however, that much more information is now available about provision of physical therapy services under IDEA and that the previous format did not lend itself to directly answering the questions that physical therapists, parents, teachers, administrators, and others continue to have. For this reason we rewrote the document using a different format.

Many people contributed to this publication. We would like to thank the following physical therapy and occupational therapy postprofessional graduate students and graduates who asked many of the questions, helped us to identify "best practices," and contributed to the content: Melanie Anderson, Becky Breaux, Sherri Cadenhead, Jennifer Campbell, Sara Cromwell, Rene Daman, Toni Doty, Bob Eskew, Kari Fields, Shawn Gable, Jeff Hammontree, Margo Hayes, Melissa Hughes, Kalpana Iyer, Leslie Jefferson, Lynn Jeffries, Maria Jones, Mary Ross Kitchen, Jana Lamb, Chris Mathews, Barbara Murphy, Megan Peters, Mary Pickett, Gary Robinson, Pam Doan Roye, Pat Pack, Sara Pellegreen, Lucy Scales, Mary Lee Stephens, Teri Collins Taylor, Joanne Walkup, and Donna Winters. Support for the students work was provided by Preparation of Related

Services Personnel grants (#H029F00056, #H029F30020, and #H029G60186) from the US Department of Education, Office of Special Education Programs, and a grant (# 6T18MC00008) from the Maternal and Child Health Bureau, Health Resources and Services Administration, US Department of Health and Human Services. Endorsement by either agency should not be inferred.

We greatly appreciate the attention to detail and suggestions provided by those who reviewed drafts of the document: Libby Gardner, Loretta Knutson, Beverly Rainforth, and Pam Roberts. Special thanks go to the Section on Pediatrics Government Affairs Committee and particularly to Susan Effgen who worked so hard to ensure that Section members had a strong voice when IDEA was reauthorized in 1997. We also thank Section members who supported the effort and waited for this update throughout the years that it took for the 1997 reauthorization and publication of the regulations in the federal Register. If we had not waited, this book would now be out of date. Thanks to Mary Jane Rapport for her contribution to the section on court decisions, letters of inquiry, and policy interpretations related to school-based physical therapy. Finally, we extend a big thanks to Nona Patten, who helps with everything and keeps us all on track.

Irene McEwen, Editor
Sandra Arnold
Maria Jones
M'Lisa Shelden

THE CARTOONS

The cartoons in this book were reprinted with the kind permission of Michael Giangreco, PhD. Michael is a good friend of related service providers and students with disabilities and their families. He is a researcher and author who contributed much of the work published on provision of related services. He also has published some of the most useful work on teamwork for inclusion of students with severe disabilities. After being involved in special education for many years, he published 3 books of cartoons[1-3] that poke gentle (and sometimes not-so-gentle) fun at the "absurdities and realities of special education." In the introduction to his second book, he commented that he wanted to be sure that people understood his beliefs, because colleagues had warned him that the cartoons could be used to promote practices that are the antithesis of what he has worked to achieve during his career. Many of his beliefs are reflected here in this document, including inclusion of students with disabilities with the necessary supports, collaborative teamwork, families as a cornerstone of educational planning, and the individualized education plan (IEP) as a powerful tool to facilitate quality education for students with disabilities. We hope that readers will see the humor in the cartoons and that they will help to promote more effective practices for children with disabilities.

REFERENCES

1. Giangreco M. Ants in His Pants: Absurdities and Realities of Special Education. Minnetonka, MN: Peytral Publications; 1998.
2. Giangreco M. Flying by the Seat of Your Pants: More Absurdities and Realities of Special Education. Minnetonka, MN: Peytral Publications; 1999.
3. Giangreco M, Ruelle K. Teaching Old Logs New Tricks: Absurdities and Realities of Education. Minnetonka, MN: Peytral Publications; 2000.

Introduction

In November 1975, the United States Congress passed Public Law 94-142.[1] The legislation was the culmination of a series of laws and court cases in the 1960s and early 1970s that increasingly defined the rights of children and adults with disabilities.[2] Part B of the Education for All Handicapped Children's Act (EHA) guaranteed the right of all children to a free and appropriate public education. Basic provisions of the act, which since the law's passage have been supported and clarified by court cases and due process hearings, include: (1) the concept of "zero reject," meaning that no children can be excluded, regardless of the severity or nature of their disabilities; (2) the concept of "least restrictive environment," meaning that children with disabilities will be educated with children who do not have disabilities to the maximum extent possible, using any necessary supplementary aids and services; (3) development of individualized education programs (IEPs) designed to meet each child's unique needs by a team that includes the child's parents; (4) provision of related services, including physical therapy, "as required to assist a [child with a disability] to benefit from special education"; and (5) the right of parents to request a due-process hearing at no cost to themselves if they disagree with their child's placement or services.[1]

Since EHA was passed over 30 years ago, many changes have occurred in how special education and physical therapy in school settings are provided. Services more often take place in natural settings, for example, instead of in isolated clinical or educational settings.[3] Exclusion and segregation of students with disabilities has been replaced by inclusion.[4] Developmentally-referenced instruction for students with severe disabilities has been replaced by functional curricula.[5] Parents have become full members of their children's educational teams.[6] These and other changes have been implemented slowly and sometimes with difficulty. Confusion and disagreement still surround many of them.

For physical therapists and other related services personnel, one of the most difficult problems has been to define appropriate public school practice. Although physical therapists were employed by a number of school districts long before EHA was implemented,[2] the practice of physical therapy in schools changed greatly under the law's mandates. The requirement that physical therapy as a related service be provided "as may be required to assist a child with a disability to benefit from special education"[1] has been one of the most controversial and confusing parts of the law, not only for therapists, but for teachers, parents, administrators, physicians, and others. Gradually, however, as research in special education and related services has been conducted and "best practices" have been described, appropriate provision of physical therapy in public schools has become clearer.[7] This document covers physical therapy services that are supported not only by the law, but also by research and contemporary practice in special education and pediatric physical therapy, which have helped to define school-based therapy.

In 1986, EHA was amended by Public Law 99-457.[8] The amendments extended special education services to children ages 3-6, and established a discretionary program (Part H) for states to provide early intervention services for infants and toddlers, from birth through 2 years of age, and their families. The individualized family service plan (IFSP) was also introduced in these amendments.

Implementation of Part H services for infants, toddlers, and their families was difficult for many professionals. In addition to requiring family-focused services instead of child-focused services that many had provided in the past, Part H mandated family involvement to: (1) establish outcomes for the child within the context of each unique family system, (2) design strategies for intervention, and (3) determine the progress that their child is making. Collaborative goal setting and program development have been easy for some professionals. Others, however, have had difficulty shifting away from an "expert" model of service provision in which professionals make most of the decisions and may impose values and priorities that conflict with those of the family. Respecting the ability of each family to make informed decisions about their child, within the context of their family structure, is a critical component of early intervention service delivery.[9]

In 1990, the law was again amended and the name was changed to the Individuals With Disabilities Education Act (IDEA).[10] IDEA added 2 eligibility categories for special education and related services: autism and traumatic brain injury. The amendment also mandated transition services for students age 16 years and older, added assistive technology and rehabilitation counseling as related services, and required state departments of education to develop policies and procedures to recruit personnel from diverse backgrounds to deliver services.

IDEA was amended in 1991 by Public Law 102-119.[11] This amendment required states to develop and implement policies and procedures needed for smooth transitions of children from early intervention to Part B programs, which provide free appropriate public education (FAPE) to children with disabilities ages 3-21.[11] It also made it possible for states to use an IFSP for children ages 3-6. Prior to these amendments, services for 3-5-year-old children needed to be identified in the more educationally oriented IEP as opposed to the more family-oriented IFSP.

In 1997 Congress passed Public Law 105-17, which further amended IDEA.[12] Some of the changes that affected physical therapy and other related services included: (1) the addition of related services to transition services; (2) the modification of the former statement that related services personnel were not required to attend IEP meetings to a statement that related services personnel should attend IEP meetings if appropriate; (3) a new provision allowing the use of IDEA funds for children with disabilities in private schools, including parochial schools; (4) an IEP focus on helping children with disabilities succeed in the general curriculum or preschool age children participate in appropriate activities; (5) increased emphasis on educating students with disabilities with students without disabilities; and (6) greater expectations for students with disabilities and agency accountability for outcomes. In addition, early intervention, which had been Part H of IDEA, became Part C.

The most recent amendment was the Individuals With Disabilities Education Improvement Act of 2004.[13] Congress further aligned IDEA with No Child Left Behind and continued to emphasize participation of children with disabilities in the general education curriculum. Some other changes of particular interest to physical therapists included: (1) a requirement that services be based on peer-reviewed research to the extent practicable; (2) changes in the requirements for individualized education program (IEP) meetings and attendance; (3) elimination of the need for short-term objectives except for students who need alternate assessment (all students must have measurable annual goals); (4) requiring transition services to be addressed when the child turns 16 years of age, rather than 14 as in IDEA 1997; and (5) giving states the option to provide early intervention services until children are kindergarten age.

Although IDEA probably is the law that has had the greatest influence on early intervention services and the education of children with disabilities, other laws also have helped to define these children's rights and opportunities. Section 504 of the Rehabilitation Act of 1973[14] and the Americans With Disabilities Act (ADA),[15] passed in 1990, are particularly important. Together, these laws give civil rights protection to people with disabilities, ensuring access to public buildings, public education, private sector employment, and all public services, accommodations, transportation, and telecommunications.

The role of physical therapists and physical therapist assistants under IDEA continues to expand and to be redefined. New legislation, ongoing litigation, and evolving definition and redefinition of effective and appropriate services for children will challenge school and early intervention teams in the future. If we can move into the future with knowledge of current laws, research, and practice, measure outcomes of the children and families we serve, and anticipate future trends and changing demands, physical therapy will continue to have an important and expanding role in early intervention and education of students with disabilities. If not, we may find it difficult to convince Congress that physical therapy should remain a part of IDEA when they amend it again in the future.

We developed this document to help physical therapy practitioners understand the provisions of IDEA that affect physical therapy practice and to apply the law in a way that is consistent with contemporary pediatric physical therapy practices and research. The document also may help other early intervention and school personnel, and families of children with disabilities to understand the provision of physical therapy services under IDEA and to learn more about current practices in pediatric physical therapy. The question and answer format of the document is intended to make it easy to find answers to the most frequent questions.

This document is not intended to provide definitive interpretation of IDEA. It also cannot cover all of the states' varying policies and procedures. For this reason, we urge physical therapy practitioners working with children who are or who might be eligible for Part C or Part B services to: (1) read 34 CFR 300 and 303, the federal regulations for IDEA; (2) obtain and read their state policy and procedures for implementation of IDEA; and (3) read peer-reviewed literature on evidence and best practices in special education and pediatric physical therapy.

The final regulations for Part B (34 CFR 300) and proposed regulations for Part C (CFR 303) are included in the compact disk (CD) that accompanies this book. At the time the book went to press in January 2009, only proposed regulations for Part C (34 CFR 303) were available. The final Part C regulations, when available, can be found at http://idea.ed.gov.

REFERENCES

1. Education for All Handicapped Children Act of 1975, 20 USC §1401 (1975).
2. Effgen SK. The educational environment. In: Campbell SK, Vander Linden DW, Palisano RJ, eds. *Physical Therapy for Children*. 3rd ed. St Louis, MO: Saunders Elsevier; 1996:955-982.
3. Rainforth B, York-Barr J. *Collaborative Teams for Students With Severe Disabilities: Integrating Therapy and Educational Services*. 2nd ed. Baltimore, MD: Paul H. Brookes; 1997.
4. Giangreco MF, Cloninger CH, Iverson VS. *Choosing Options and Accommodations for Children: A Guide to Educational Planning for Students with Disabilities*. 2nd ed. Baltimore, MD: Paul H. Brookes; 1998.
5. Harris SR. Functional abilities in context. In: Lister MJ, ed. *Contemporary Management of Motor Control Problems: Proceedings of the II STEP Conference*. Alexandria, VA: Foundation for Physical Therapy; 1991: 253-259.
6. Turnbull AP, Turnbull HR. *Families, Professionals, and Exceptity: A Special Partnership*. 2nd ed. Upper Saddle River, NJ: Prentice-Hall; 1997.
7. McEwen IR, Shelden ML. Pediatric physical therapy in the 1990s: the demise of the educational versus medical dichotomy. *Phys Occup Ther Pediatr.* 1995;15(2):33-45.
8. Education of the Handicapped Amendments of 1986, 20 U.S.C. §1401.
9. Rosin P, Whitehead AD, Tuchman LI, Jesein GS, Begun AL, Irwin L. *Partnerships in Family Centered Care: A Guide to Collaborative Early Intervention*. Baltimore, MD: Paul H. Brookes; 1996.
10. Individuals With Disabilities Education Act of 1990, 20 USC §1401 (1990).
11. Individuals With Disabilities Education Act Amendments of 1991, 20 USC §1401 (1991).
12. Individuals With Disabilities Education Act Amendments of 1997, 20 USC §1401 (1997).
13. Individuals With Disabilities Education Act Amendments of 2004, 20 USC §1401 (2004).
14. Rehabilitation Act of 1973 §504, 29 USC §794 (1973).
15. Americans With Disabilities Act of 1990, 42 USC §12101 (1990).

Section I: Questions & Answers

The Code of Federal Regulations 34 (34 CFR) Parts 300 and 303 are regulations for the Individuals With Disabilities Education Act (IDEA) and are included in the CD that accompanies this book. Part 300 covers Part B of IDEA (education of children with disabilities) and Part 303 covers Part C (early intervention programs for infants and toddlers with disabilities). Because physical therapy practitioners working under the provisions of IDEA need to know and understand the regulations, we have quoted (in italics) and referenced sections of 34 CFR 300 or the proposed Section 303 throughout this document. We encourage readers to refer to these sources for more complete information on each topic and for information on topics not covered. Because the final Part C regulations (34 CFR 303) were not available when this book went to press, the content related to Part C is based on the proposed regulations. Check http://idea.ed.gov when the final Part C regulations are available to see if any changes were made.

Prior to the regulations becoming final, the US Department of Education held public hearings and solicited comments about a draft of the regulations. The Federal Register with the final regulations includes many pages of analyses of comments received by along with the Department of Education's responses to the comments. The "Analysis of Comments and Changes" section, which precedes the regulations, is organized by section and subsection of the regulations and gives a wealth of information to help interpret them.

1 Employment of Physical Therapists Under IDEA

Irene McEwen, PT, PhD, FAPTA

This chapter covers qualifications and other employment-related considerations for physical therapists providing services under IDEA and their employers.

What are the requirements to be a "highly qualified" physical therapist?

IDEA 2004 aligns with No Child Left Behind (NCLB) to require special education teachers to be "highly qualified," as defined by NCLB. The law does not use the term "highly qualified" for physical therapists and other related services providers, or for early intervention personnel.

Does the law say anything about qualifications of physical therapists?

Under Part B, qualifications of physical therapists and other related services providers are addressed under Sec. 300.156 Personal qualifications (a-b):

- *(a) General. The SEA (State Education Agency) must establish and maintain qualifications to ensure that personnel necessary to carry out the purposes of this part are appropriately and adequately prepared and trained, including that those personnel have the content knowledge and skills to serve children with disabilities.*
- *(b) Related services personnel and paraprofessionals. The qualifications under paragraph (a) of this section must include qualifications for related services personnel and paraprofessionals that—*
  - *(1) Are consistent with any State-approved or State-recognized certification, licensing, registration, or other comparable requirements that apply to the professional discipline in which those personnel are providing special education or related services; and*
  - *(2) Ensure that related services personnel who deliver services in their discipline or profession—*
    - *(i) Meet the requirements of paragraph (b)(1) of this section; and*
    - *(ii) Have not had certification or licensure requirements waived on an emergency, temporary, or provisional basis; and*
    - *(iii) Allow paraprofessionals and assistants who are appropriately trained and supervised, in accordance with State law, regulation, or written policy, in meeting the requirements of this part to be used to assist in the provision of special education and related services under this part to children with disabilities.*

IDEA 1997 required professionals to meet the highest standards of a State, but IDEA 2004 removed this requirement. In the Analysis of Comments and Changes section of the Federal Register prior to the regulations for Part B (see the CD with this book), the U.S. Department of Education responded to concerns, particularly from speech-language pathologists, about this change, saying:

> *We are not changing Sec. 300.156 because it reflects the specific language in section 612(a)(14) of the Act, which was intended to provide greater flexibility to SEAs to establish appropriate personnel standards, including the standards for speech-language pathologists. As indicated in note 97 of the Conf. Rpt., p. 192, section 612(a)(14) of the Act removes the requirement for State professional requirements to be based on the highest requirements in the State because of concerns that the previous law, regarding the qualifications of related services providers, established an unreasonable standard for SEAs to meet, and as a result, led to a shortage of related services providers for children with disabilities. We believe that States can exercise the flexibility provided in Sec. 300.156 and section 612(a)(14) of the Act while ensuring appropriate services for children with disabilities without additional regulation.* (71 FR 46610)

The term "highly qualified" is not used in Part C. Physical therapists and other personnel must be "qualified," as defined in Sec. 303.31:

> *Qualified personnel means personnel who have met State approved or recognized certification, licensing, registration, or other comparable requirements that apply to the area in which the individuals are providing early intervention services.*

What are qualifications for physical therapists?

All physical therapists must have graduated from an accredited professional (entry-level) physical therapist education program and be licensed in the state or states in which they practice.[1] Depending largely on when a physical therapist graduated, the professional credential could be a bachelor's, master's, or doctoral degree, or a postbaccalaureate certificate. Since 2002, the Commission on Accreditation in Physical Therapy Education (CAPTE) has accredited only programs that award a postbaccalaureate degree. Physical therapists who graduated from accredited programs with bachelor's degrees continue to be eligible for licensure. Currently, the majority of physical therapist education programs in the United States award a professional doctor of physical therapy (DPT) degree.

Physical therapists who graduated from programs outside the United States that were not accredited by CAPTE must have their credentials evaluated and determined to be equivalent to professional preparation of accredited programs in the United States. States also may have other requirements for physical therapists educated outside the United States.

Many physical therapists have additional qualifications, such as advanced practice postprofessional degrees and certification as clinical specialists through the American Board of Physical Therapy Specialties. Most clinical specialists working in schools have Pediatric Clinical Specialist (PCS) certification. Physical therapists may also have other types of certifications and credentials, such as Assistive Technology Provider (ATP) certification.

What are the requirements for licensure?

Physical therapy is regulated as a health care profession at the state level. Every state in the United States has a practice act for physical therapists and regulations for administering the state law. The Web site of the Federation of State Boards of Physical Therapy at www.fsbpt.org provides information about the authority in each state, contact information, and links to the practice act and other information. In most states the license must be renewed annually for a fee, and many states require evidence of continuing competence through relevant educational activities, such as continuing education courses, postprofessional university coursework, teaching, and writing for publication.

Are additional qualifications necessary to work under IDEA?

In addition to licensure as a physical therapist, some state education agencies have established generic and specific standards for certification of professionals working in the public and private schools. Other states have certification for early intervention service providers. Requirements vary by state and the certification process may have various levels (emergency, initial, continuing) and specific regulations related to issuance, renewal, and reinstatement.

Even when states do not require certification to work in early intervention or schools, physical therapists usually need knowledge and skills beyond their physical therapist education programs to work appropriately and effectively with children with disabilities under IDEA.[2,3] Physical therapist education programs must prepare students to be competent generalists, capable of working in any environment, such as hospitals, extended care facilities, rehabilitation centers for adults, and outpatient orthopedic clinics, with people of all ages. Few programs teach much, if anything, about working with children with disabilities and their families under IDEA, probably because fewer than 5% of all physical therapists work in schools, according to surveys by the American Physical Therapy Association.[4] The surveys did not address early intervention, and the percentage of physical therapists who work in early intervention programs is not known.

What additional information do physical therapists need to work with children with disabilities and their families under IDEA?

Competencies for physical therapists working in early intervention programs[2] and providing school-based services[3] have been published as personnel standards for therapists, educators, administrators, and consumers to monitor the quality of service delivery. An essential competency that crosses early intervention and school-based practice is knowledge of relevant local, state, and federal laws, rules, and regulations. Without this knowledge, no one can provide appropriate and effective services. Competent physical therapists may not have achieved all of the other competencies, but they should serve as a guideline for individual personnel development.[2,3]

Tables 1-1 and 1-2 list the competencies for early intervention and school-based practice, respectively. The articles in which the competencies were published[2,3] give additional information about each of them and activities under each area. Some of the competencies are specific to physical therapy, but many are generic, necessary for professionals of any discipline working with children and their families under IDEA.

Do physical therapists need a physician's referral to work with children under IDEA?

Physical therapists working with children under IDEA must comply with their state practice acts. In the majority of states, children have direct access to physical therapy and a referral is not necessary, unless required by school district policy or for reimbursement. In some states without direct access for all patients, a referral is not required for physical therapy provided under IDEA. Some states also allow evaluation, but not intervention, without a referral. The Web site of the Federation of State Boards of Physical Therapy at www.fsbpt.org provides links to the practice acts of each state.

How often must medical referrals be obtained?

In states without direct access, a "current" medical referral usually is required, which may be interpreted differently from state to state. Generally, if no definition of "current" exists, an annual referral is considered current.

What if a medical referral is not consistent with the team's decision about the type of therapy, frequency, and/or duration?

A medical referral is just one piece of input to the child's individualized family service plan (IFSP) or individualized education program (IEP) team. The team must consider every team member's input, within the context of the child's overall program. Neither a physician nor any other team member can make decisions in isolation.[5] If a physician's referral specifies a type or intensity of physical therapy that is inconsistent with the decisions of the rest of the team, then a team member (usually the physical therapist or parent) must contact the physician and resolve the differences. The referral cannot be ignored; but neither can the physician order the physical therapy to be provided.

Table 1-1. Early-Intervention Competency Areas

Content Area A: The context of therapy in early intervention settings

1. Demonstrate knowledge of local, state, and federal laws, rules, and regulations regarding service delivery
   a) *discuss the implications of PL 94–142, PL 99–457, PL 105–17, and PL 108–446 and their reauthorizations*
   b) *apply the guidelines of federal, state and local regulations*
   c) *identify and use information sources for federal, state, and local legislation and regulation changes*
   d) *discuss and demonstrate professional behavior regarding ethical and legal responsibilities*
   e) *discuss professional competencies as defined by professional organizations and state regulations*
   f) *advocate to support family and child entitlements*
2. Demonstrate knowledge of family systems theory, recognize the central importance of the family, and be able to provide family-centered services
   a) *identify and discuss how the following factors may affect a child's and family's experience with an early intervention program:*
      i. *cultural*
      ii. *socioeconomic*
      iii. *ethical*
      iv. *historical*
      v. *personal values*
   b) *conduct a family interview using active listening skills to gather information on: family's knowledge, strengths, concerns, and priorities regarding their*
      i. *child*
      ii. *family lifestyle and beliefs*
      iii. *services and outcomes desired*
   c) *respect the family and acknowledge that the family is the most significant member of the team*
   d) *advocate that children are best understood in the contexts of family, culture, and community*
3. Recognize the impact of a child with special needs on a family unit throughout the family life cycle
   a) *describe a typical daily routine and activities that families may encounter*
   b) *implement basic strategies to support the family unit, including the parents, parent-child relationships, and sibling subsystems*
4. Support the parents' primary roles as mother and father to the child
   a) *assist the family in identifying and developing:*
      i. *internal and external resources*
      ii. *a social support network*
      iii. *advocacy skills*
   b) *advocate the right of parents to be decision makers in the early intervention process*
   c) *provide parents with the information and options needed for informed decisions*
   d) *respect parents' choices and goals for their children*
5. Collaborate and encourage family involvement with the early-intervention process
   a) *implement, a range of family-oriented services based on the family's identified resources, priorities, and concerns*
   b) *provide information on family oriented conferences and support groups in the community*
   c) *demonstrate people first and family friendly communication and interaction skills*
   d) *communicate effectively with parents about curriculum and the child's progress*

Content Area B: Wellness and prevention in early intervention settings

1. Promote public awareness of early-intervention services
   a) *disseminate information about the availability, criteria for eligibility, and methods of referral*
   b) *collect and use data from multiple sources for child-find systems*

Table 1-1. Early-Intervention Competency Areas (continued)

2. Design and implement a screening program to identify infants and toddlers at risk for developmental delay:
   a) *demonstrate knowledge of genetic and cultural differences in standards of growth and development*
   b) *identify the etiology, signs and symptoms, and classifications of common pediatric disabilities*
   c) *identify established biological and environmental factors that affect children's development and learning*
   d) *demonstrate understanding of developmental consequences of maternal health and nutrition, social supports, and stress*
3. Select, administer, and interpret a variety of screening instruments and standardized measurement tools: *Apply knowledge of:*
   a) *child development from cognitive, adaptive, motor, social-emotional, and communication perspectives*
   b) *the interrelationship among developmental areas*
   c) *the range of normal variations of development*
   d) *the difference between delayed and atypical development*
4. Promote child safety by educating caregivers on:
   a) *child development*
   b) *environmental and toy hazards and safety measures*
   c) *accident prevention*
   d) *recognition of child neglect and abuse*

Content Area C: Coordinated care in early intervention settings

1. Form a partnership and work collaboratively with other team members, especially the child's family:
   a) *refer and coordinate services among family, other professionals, community agencies, day care programs*
   b) *demonstrate effective and appropriate interpersonal communication skills*
   c) *implement strategies for team development and management*
   d) *develop mechanism for ongoing team coordination*
   e) *function as an interdisciplinary or transdisciplinary team member*
   f) *if applicable, serve as a service coordinator*
2. Function as a consultant:
   a) *identify the administrative and interpersonal factors that influence the effectiveness of a consultant*
   b) *provide technical assistance to other early intervention team members, community agencies, and medical facilities*
3. Supervise personnel and professional students:
   a) *monitor the implementation of therapy recommendations by other team members*
   b) *establish a student clinical affiliation*
   c) *formally and informally teach/train therapy staff*

Content Area D: Evaluation and assessment in the early intervention setting

1. Individualize the evaluation and assessment for child, team, and family needs:
   a) *offer flexible scheduling*
   b) *provide options for multiple settings*
   c) *solicit input on the process*
   d) *establish consensus of content including domains of child development and family routines*
2. Evaluate family strengths, resources, concerns, and priorities:
   a) *conduct family interview*
   b) *select and administer supplemental family surveys*
3. Selectively gather, interpret, and report information from available medical/developmental records
4. Evaluate and assess child abilities and strengths including:
   a) *functional ability including activities of daily living, play, and gross motor, fine motor, perceptual motor, and oral motor skills*
   b) *musculoskeletal status*
   c) *neuromotor status*

Table 1-1. Early-Intervention Competency Areas (continued)

- *d) sensory status*
- *e) cardiopulmonary status*

5. Use valid, reliable, and nondiscriminatory examination instruments and procedures for:
    - *a) identification and eligibility*
    - *b) diagnostic evaluation*
    - *c) individual program planning*
    - *d) documentation of child progress, family outcomes, and program impact*
6. Function as a team leader and/or member in a multidisciplinary, interdisciplinary, or transdisciplinary assessment through:
    - *a) organization*
    - *b) time management*
    - *c) timeliness*
    - *d) constructive feedback*
    - *e) consensus building*
    - *f) wrap-up*

Content Area E: Planning

1. Actively participate in the development of the Individualized Family Service Plan (IFSP):
    - *a) accurately interpret and communicate examination findings to the family and other team members*
    - *b) discuss and integrate examination findings from family and other team members*
    - *c) solicit from family their goals of the early intervention process*
    - *d) Prioritize needs identified during examination according to:*
        - *i. family preference and goals*
        - *ii. environmental demand*
        - *iii. future environmental demands*
        - *iv. resources*
        - *v. developmental level*
        - *vi. past history*
    - *e) collaboratively establish IFSP outcomes that are meaningful to the child and family*
    - *f) communicate options for strategies, programs and services to family*
    - *g) establish consensus on strategies, programs and services*
2. Integrate an interdisciplinary understanding of the home, child care, medical and social community of the child and family into the IFSP:
    - *a) inquire about family routines and activities*
    - *b) establish contact and with permission consult with child care / preschool providers*
    - *c) establish collaborative relationship with any relevant medical personnel*
    - *d) inquire about community resources from local interagency coordinating council*
    - *e) gather family information on community activities, programs, services, and resources*
3. Develop mechanism for ongoing coordination and collaboration regarding the IFSP:
    - *a) implementation of the IFSP*
    - *b) update or modify IFSP*
    - *c) transition planning and implementation of the transition plan*
    - *d) interagency activities*

Content Area F: Intervention

1. Develop and implement appropriate intervention programs and strategies that address or incorporate:
    - *a) self-care, mobility, learning and play*
    - *b) values of the family and child's culture*
    - *c) developmentally and individually appropriate activities*
    - *d) environmental adaptations in the home and community*

Table 1-1. Early-Intervention Competency Areas (continued)

- *e) information and strategies from multiple disciplines*
- *f) medical care of infants and toddlers*
- *g) methods of behavior support and management*

2. Assist families in accessing services that promote full inclusion of child and family into the community:
   - *a) provide services in the child's natural environments*
   - *b) communicate with, and educate, family/caregivers, teachers, and others regarding intervention strategies*
   - *c) implement small group parent-child and peer activities when appropriate for a particular community setting*
   - *d) link current intervention plan with the next educational setting*
3. Integrate therapy intervention strategies into home and community settings:
   - *a) support and facilitate family child interaction as primary context for learning and development*
   - *b) use daily routines including child care activities such as feeding, bathing, dressing, and playing*
   - *c) use parent and child mediated activities during intervention*
   - *d) modify intervention strategies according to changes in the child's interests, functional level, medical status, or family needs*

Content Area G: Documentation issues in early-intervention settings

1. Produce useful written documentation by:
   - *a) using commonly understood and meaningful terms*
   - *b) maintaining timely and consistent records*
   - *c) concisely summarizing relevant information*
   - *d) sharing records with family and other team members*
2. Demonstrate the ability to write the IFSP document, including:
   - *a) current developmental and functional status of the child*
   - *b) long-and short-term child and family objectives that are meaningful, functional and measurable*
   - *c) objective means of monitoring progress*
   - *d) description of the early intervention and community services*
   - *e) justification for frequency, intensity, location, and service delivery*
3. Document to convey information to family, other team members, and funding agencies, including:
   - *a) summary of intervention session*
   - *b) child's response*
   - *c) ideas for daily activities and routines*
   - *d) plans for new intervention strategies and resources*
4. Collaboratively monitor and modify child's intervention plan:
   - *a) establish a mechanism for ongoing communication with family and other team members*
   - *b) record summary of communications with family and other team members*
   - *c) establish a plan for re-evaluation*
   - *d) schedule pre-established team meetings to review child's progress*
5. Evaluate and document the effectiveness of therapy intervention strategies and therapeutic procedures:
   - *a) establish baseline of child's developmental and functional status*
   - *b) collect ongoing data on the child's progress toward stated IFSP outcomes*
   - *c) summarize data to determine child's progress*
   - *d) make recommendations for modifications of IFSP*

Content Area H: Administration issues in early intervention settings

1. Function as an administrator:
   - *a) identify the philosophy, goals, structure and function, and administrative needs of the early intervention program and therapy services*
   - *b) apply knowledge of other disciplines' roles and functions for program planning and policy formation*

Table 1-1. Early-Intervention Competency Areas (continued)

c) *develop and implement criteria and procedures for job descriptions, recruitment, staff selection, supervision, and performance appraisals*
d) *develop therapy policies and procedures*
e) *direct therapy services and delegate appropriate responsibilities*
f) *establish appropriate and manageable caseloads*
g) *meet deadlines in order to be able to provide services in a timely and efficient manner*
h) *identify and develop appropriate referral mechanisms*
i) *develop procedures for documenting service in accordance with Codes of Ethics, funding agency policies, and federal, state, and local regulations*

2. Demonstrate the ability to assist and support the professional development of early intervention personnel:
   a) *identify and access intramural and extramural funding sources and resources*
      i. *community*
      ii. *state*
      iii. *national*
   b) *provide onsite inservice training*
   c) *establish intra-agency mentoring program*
   d) *implement individualized professional development plan*
3. Demonstrate leadership abilities in promoting effective team processes:
   a) *facilitate regularly scheduled staff meetings*
   b) *implement mentor program*
   c) *provide opportunity for staff inservice trainings*
   d) *selectively delegate responsibilities*
   e) *allocate time for team collaboration*
   f) *mediate team differences*

Content Area I: Research in early intervention settings

1. Demonstrate knowledge of current research relating to infant development, medical care, and developmental intervention for infants and toddlers:
   a) *conduct a literature review using such reference materials as Index Medicus, or other data base sources*
   b) *seek assistance from experienced researchers in interpreting published research*
   c) *critically evaluate published research*
2. Apply knowledge of research to the selection of therapy intervention strategies, service delivery systems, and therapeutic procedures in early intervention:
   a) *use objective criteria for evaluation*
   b) *justify rationale for clinical decision making*
   c) *expand clinical cases into single-subject studies*
3. Partake in program evaluation and clinical research activities with the appropriate supervision:
   a) *identify topics in early intervention in which research efforts are needed*
   b) *secure resources to support clinical research*
   c) *implement clinical research projects*
   d) *disseminate research findings*

(Reprinted from Chiarello L and Effgen S. Updated Competencies for physical therapists working in early intervention. *Pediatr Phys Ther.* 2006;18:151-154, with permission from Lippincott Williams & Wilkins and the Section on Pediatrics of the American Physical Therapy Association.)

Table 1-2. Competencies for School-Based Therapists

Content Area 1: The context of therapy practice in schools

1. Knowledge of the structure, global goals, and responsibilities of the public education system, including special education:
   a) *diagram the functional and supervisory organization of the education system served by the therapist*
   b) *identify the goals and outcomes of the educational curriculum from preschool through high school*
   c) *demonstrate an understanding of the eventual goals of independent living and working*
   d) *apply knowledge of the outcomes-based education curriculum*
2. Knowledge of federal (for example IDEA, Rehabilitation Act of 1973, and ADA), state, and local laws and regulations that affect the delivery of services to students with disabilities:
   a) *discuss the implications of the laws (national, state, and local)*
   b) *apply the guidelines of federal, state, and local regulations*
   c) *identify and use information sources for federal, state, and local legislation and regulation changes*
   d) *discuss and demonstrate professional behavior regarding ethical and legal responsibilities*
   e) *discuss professional competencies as defined by professional organizations and state regulations*
   f) *advocate to support services related to educational entitlements*
3. Knowledge of the theoretical and functional orientation of a variety of professionals serving students within the educational system:
   a) *initiate dialogue with colleagues to exchange professional perspectives*
   b) *disseminate information about the availability of therapy services, criteria for eligibility, and methods of referral*
   c) *describe evaluations and interventions commonly used by psychologists, diagnostic educators, classroom teachers, speech and language pathologists, adaptive physical educators, nurses, physical therapists, occupational therapists, and professionals in other education and health-related disciplines*
4. Assist students in accessing community organizations, resources, and activities:
   a) *demonstrate awareness of cultural and social differences that relate to family and student participation in the education program*
   b) *in collaboration with the educational team, develop a plan for transition into community activities or adult services*
   c) *identify the need to make appropriate student referrals to community therapy and recreational services when school services are not able to meet all of the child's needs*
   d) *include the family in the educational process*
   e) *serve as a resource to family and other team members for information and appropriate community resources (medical, educational, financial, social, recreational, and legal)*

Content Area 2: Wellness and prevention in schools

1. Implement school-wide screening program with school nurses, physical education teachers, and teachers:
   a) *apply knowledge of risk factors affecting growth, development, and learning*
   b) *identify the etiology, signs, symptoms, and classifications of common pediatric disabilities*
   c) *identify established biological and environmental factors that affect children's development and learning*
   d) *select, administer, and interpret a variety of screening instruments and standardized measurement tools*
2. Promote child safety and wellness using knowledge of environmental safety measures:
   a) *maintain CPR certification*
   b) *institute an environmental hazards and accident prevention plan*
   c) *recognize child neglect and abuse*

Content Area 3: Team collaboration

1. Form partnerships and work collaboratively with other team members, especially the teacher to promote an effective plan of care:
   a) *demonstrate effective communication and interpersonal skills*

Table 1-2. Competencies for School-Based Therapists (continued)

- *b) refer and coordinate services among family, school professionals, medical service providers, and community agencies*
- *c) implement strategies for team development and management*
- *d) develop mechanism for ongoing team coordination*

2. Function as a consultant:
   - *a) identify the administrative and interpersonal factors that influence the effectiveness of a consultant*
   - *b) implement effective consultative strategies*
   - *c) provide technical assistance to other school team members, community agencies, and medical providers*
3. Educate school personnel and family to promote the inclusion of the student within the educational experience:
   - *a) assist school administrators with development of policy and procedures*
   - *b) provide orientation to teachers and classroom aides*
   - *c) conduct in-service sessions*
   - *d) develop informational resources*
4. Supervise personnel and professional students:
   - *a) apply effective strategies of supervision*
   - *b) monitor the implementation of therapy recommendations by other team members*
   - *c) establish a student clinical affiliation*
   - *d) formally and informally teach or train therapy staff*
5. Serve as an advocate for students, families, and school:
   - *a) attend public hearings*
   - *b) serve on task forces or decision-making committees*
   - *c) provide necessary information to support student rights*
   - *d) actively participate in IEP process*

Content Area 4: Examination and evaluation in schools

1. Identify strengths and needs of students:
   - *a) interview student, family, teachers, and other relevant school personnel*
   - *b) gather information from medical personnel and records*
   - *c) observe student in a variety of educational settings*
2. Collaboratively determine examination and evaluation process:
   - *a) designate appropriate professional disciplines*
   - *b) identify environments and student activities and routines*
   - *c) select instruments*
   - *d) establish format for conducting examination*
   - *e) inform and prepare the student*
3. Determine student's ability to participate in meaningful school activities by examining and evaluating:
   - *a) level of participation and necessary assistance and adaptations through formal naturalistic observations*
   - *b) functional abilities including gross motor, fine motor, perceptual motor, cognitive, social and emotional, and ADL*
   - *c) impairments related to functional ability including musculoskeletal status, neuromotor organization, sensory function, and cardiopulmonary status*
4. Utilize valid, reliable, cost-effective, and nondiscriminatory instruments for:
   - *a) identification and eligibility*
   - *b) diagnostic purposes*
   - *c) individual program planning*
   - *d) documentation of progress*

Content Area 5: Planning

1. Actively participate in the development of the Individualized Education Plan:

Table 1-2. Competencies for School-Based Therapists (continued)

- *a) determine eligibility related to a student's educational program*
- *b) accurately interpret and communicate examination findings collaboratively with family, student, and other team members*
- *c) discuss prognosis of student performance related to curricular expectations*
- *d) discuss and prioritize outcomes related to student's educational needs based on current and future environmental demands and student and family preferences and goals*
- *e) offer appropriate recommendations for student placement and personnel needs in the least restrictive educational setting with intent to serve children in inclusive environments*
- *f) in collaboration with the team, determine how therapy can contribute to the development of an individualized educational program (IEP) including*
  - *i. meaningful student outcomes*
  - *ii. functional and measurable goals and objectives*
  - *iii. therapy service recommendations*
  - *iv. specific intervention methods and strategies*
  - *v. determination of frequency, intensity, and duration*
- *g) develop mechanism for ongoing coordination and collaboration regarding the IEP*
  - *i. implementation of the IEP*
  - *ii. updating or modifying IEP*
  - *iii. transition planning and implementation of the transition plan*
  - *iv. interagency activities*

Content Area 6: Intervention

1. Adapt environments to facilitate student access to and participation in student activities:
   - *a) recommend adaptive equipment, assistive technology, and environmental adaptations*
   - *b) monitor adaptive equipment, assistive technology, and environmental adaptations*
   - *c) be able to instruct student and other team members in the appropriate use of adaptive equipment and assistive technology*
   - *d) identify sources for obtaining, maintaining, repairing, and financing adaptive equipment, assistive technology, and environmental adaptations*
2. Use various types and methods of service provision for individualized student interventions:
   - *a) direct, individual, group, integrated, consultative, monitoring, and collaborative approaches*
   - *b) develop generic instruction plans and intervention plans that select and sequence strategies to meet the objectives listed on the student's IEP*
3. Promote skill acquisition, fluency, and generalization to enhance overall development, learning, and student participation:
   - *a) use creative problem-solving strategies to meet the student's needs*
   - *b) explain basic motor learning theories, and relate them to therapy education programs*
   - *c) address neuromuscular, musculoskeletal, sensory processing, and cardiopulmonary functions that support motor, social, emotional, cognitive, and language skills*
4. Imbed therapy interventions into the context of student activities and routines:
   - *a) implement appropriate positioning, mobility, environmental, and ADL strategies into curriculum, classroom schedule and routines*
   - *b) develop a matrix integrating objectives, routines and activities, and strategies*

Content Area 7: Documentation

1. Produce useful written documentation by:
   - *a) writing reports in commonly understood and meaningful terms*
   - *b) maintaining timely and consistent records*
   - *c) concisely summarizing relevant information*
   - *d) sharing records with family and other team members*
2. Collaboratively monitor and modify student's IEP
   - *a) establish a mechanism for and record ongoing communication with family and other team members*

Table 1-2. Competencies for School-Based Therapists (continued)

   b) *establish a plan of action for reevaluation*
   c) *schedule pre-established team meetings to review student progress over the course of the school year*
3. Evaluate and document the effectiveness of therapy programs:
   a) *establish baseline of student's level of participation and functional status*
   b) *collect ongoing data on the student's progress toward stated IEP outcomes*
   c) *summarize data to determine student's progress*

Content Area 8: Administrative issues in schools

1. Demonstrate flexibility, priority setting, and effective time management strategies
2. Obtain resources and data necessary to justify establishing a new therapy program or altering an existing program
3. Serve as a leader:
   a) *integrate knowledge of education, health, and social trends that impact therapy services*
   b) *identify and educate others about the overall roles, responsibilities, and functions of therapy services*
   c) *identify and differentiate characteristics of alternative approaches for resolving needs for therapy services*
   d) *identify the administrative needs of the therapy service within the school setting*
   e) *serve as a role model to other therapists regarding professional responsibilities*
4. Serve as a manager:
   a) *develop and analyze job descriptions for therapists*
   b) *implement a recruitment, orientation, mentorship, and professional development program for therapists and staff*
   c) *develop and implement policies and procedures to guide therapy services*
   d) *establish therapy caseloads and staffing needs*
   e) *evaluate the performance of therapy personnel*
   f) *plan and implement a therapy quality assurance plan and program evaluation*
   g) *participate in the assessment of school facilities and educational activities*
   h) *make recommendations, especially related to ensuring accessibility to and reasonable accommodations in school environments*
   i) *identify and use appropriate school, home, community, state, and national resources, especially funding sources*
   j) *demonstrate the ability to plan and manage a budget for the therapy component of services*

Content Area 9: Research

1. Demonstrate knowledge of current research relating to child development, medical care, educational practices, and implications for therapy:
   a) *conduct a literature review*
   b) *seek assistance from experienced researchers in interpreting published research*
   c) *critically evaluate published research*
2. Apply knowledge of research to the selection of therapy intervention strategies, service delivery systems, and therapeutic procedures:
   a) *use objective criteria for evaluation*
   b) *justify rationale for clinical decision making*
   c) *expand clinical treatment case reports into single-subject studies*
3. Partake in program evaluation and clinical research activities with the appropriate supervision:
   a) *identify research topics*
   b) *secure resources to support clinical research*
   c) *implement clinical research projects*
   d) *disseminate research findings*

(Reprinted from Effgen SK, Chiarello LA, Milbourne SA. Updated competencies for physical therapists working in schools. *Pediatr Phys Ther.* 2007;19:269-271, with permission from Lippincott Williams & Wilkins and the Section on Pediatrics of the American Physical Therapy Association.)

Table 1-3. Considerations When Determining a Physical Therapist's Caseload

The students to be served	Considerations should include the type and amount of assessment and intervention needed by each student, the geographic area to be covered by the physical therapist, the number of schools to be covered, and the travel time between schools.
The physical therapist's other identified responsibilities	In addition to evaluation and intervention with students, responsibilities may include keeping records, attending and reporting at student-related and other meetings, consultation with parents and school personnel, and assessing the need for equipment, scheduling, conducting needs assessment, conducting outcome studies, and supervisory responsibilities.
Other factors related to provision of service	Other factors to consider include: 1. The amount of consultation required by the teacher and other classroom staff and school personnel; 2. The amount of consultation required by parents; 3. The amount of support available from aides, assistants, and clerical personnel; 4. Students' needed for one-to-one intervention as opposed to group intervention; 5. The number of community contacts required with other agencies and professionals; and 6. The amount of continuing education the physical therapist needs to achieve or maintain competence.

Adapted with permission from: Martin KD, ed. *Physical Therapy Practice in Educational Environments: Policies and Guidelines.* Alexandria, Va: American Physical Therapy Association; 1990.

How many children make up a full-time caseload?

The number of children in a physical therapist's caseload depends on many things, and no federal regulations address the size of a caseload. State or local guidelines may exist and reflect unique features of service delivery, considering such things as: the number of homes, schools, or other locations in which a therapist must provide service; the distances between locations; the number of evaluations the therapist is expected to perform; the experience of the therapist and other personnel; the administrative and/or supervisory activities of the therapist; the number of support personnel available; the needs of the children and families; and the availability of other therapists. Table 1-3 lists these and other considerations for determining case loads and Table 1-4 illustrates use of a time-log analysis to determine caseloads in a school district.[6]

SUMMARY

Physical therapists are licensed health professionals whose practices are regulated by state law. Practice acts vary from state to state, making knowledge of the practice act of the state in which a physical therapist practices important. The Website of the Federation of State Boards of Physical Therapy at www.fsbpt.org is a good source of information about physical therapy licensure and has links to the practice acts of each state and other US jurisdictions. Some states have requirements in addition to licensure for physical therapists to work in schools or early intervention, such as certification or other type of credential.

Table 1-4. Time-Log Analysis to Determine Caseload

The amount of time available for examination, direct treatment, and monitoring classroom programs may vary from one setting to another.

The school year calendar may also cause variety. However, the following is a breakdown of the average time consumed in a physical therapist's typical week from two perspectives:

1. Percentage of time spent by the physical therapist in various activities

Total working hours per week—FTE physical therapist (taken from Tacoma Public Schools caseload survey, February 1986)

		Itinerant PT	*School-based PT*
Contract conditions*	(20%)	7.50 hrs	7.50 hrs (20%)
Student contact	(44%)	16.50 hrs	17.30 hrs (46%)
Paperwork	(14%)	5.25 hrs	4.90 hrs (13%)
Meeting, IEP	(11%)	4.10 hrs	7.80 hrs (21%)
Travel	(11%)	4.10 hrs	0.00 hrs
Total		37.50 hrs	37.50 hrs

*Contract conditions:

Lunch time	2.5 hrs
Breaks	2.5 hrs
Planning time	2.5 hrs
Total	7.5 hrs

2. Balance of time for treatment after subtracting required activities

Total working hours per week—37.5 (taken from Michigan Alliance of School PTs and OTs, March 1986)

Assessment	2.5 hrs
Documentation, planning, preparation	2.5 hrs
IEP staffings and meetings	2.5 hrs
Consultation	2.0 hrs
Lunch	2.5 hrs
Balance (intervention time)	25.5 hrs

Clearly, these hours are theoretically available, but do not include what is actually available to any given physical therapist. There are innumerable variables, such as travel time, scheduling conflicts, liaison work with community resources, student assessments, supervisory responsibility, inservices to staff, etc. These variables directly influence the time actually available for student contact.

In summary, caseload numbers can be determined by examining both the categorization of student needs and the amount of time actually available to fulfill the IEP recommendations. In both these examples, the student contact time on intervention time is the time sued to calculate caseload.

Reprinted from "Guidelines for Physical Therapy Practice in Educational Environments of Washington State." Olympic, Wash. Pediatric Special Interest Group, Washington State Physical Therapy Association; 1987 with permission from the Washington State Physical Therapy Association.

REFERENCES

1. *Guide to Physical Therapist Practice*. Revised 2nd ed. Alexandria, VA: American Physical Therapy Association; 2003.
2. Chiarello L, Effgen S. Updated competencies for physical therapists working in early intervention. *Pediatr Phys Ther.* 2006;18:148-158.
3. Effgen SK, Chiarello LA, Milbourne SA. Updated competencies for physical therapists working in schools. *Pediatr Phys Ther.* 2007;19:266-274.
4. American Physical Therapy Association Web site. Physical therapist member demographic profile 1996–2006. http://www.apta.org/AM/Template.cfm?Section=Surveys_and_Stats1&Template=/MembersOnly.cfm&ContentID=38175. Accessed June 12, 2007.
5. Okamoto GA, McEwen IR, Marlowe K, Hammons G. Prescriptions for physical and occupational therapy in school. *Arch Phys Med Rehabil.* 1983;64:429-31.
6. Martin KD, ed. *Physical Therapy Practice in Educational Environment: Policies and Guidelines.* Alexandria, VA: American Physical Therapy Association; 1990.

2 Understanding and Strengthening Parental Involvement

Elizabeth DeGrace, PhD, OTR/L, and Traci Castles, BS

Parent involvement is a familiar concept for those working in early intervention programs or school systems. When parents are involved in their child's early intervention or education programs, common sense tells us that their involvement will positively influence child outcomes. Indeed, a synthesis of research related to parental involvement found:

> *... the evidence is consistent, positive, and convincing: families have a major influence on their children's achievement in school and through life. When schools, families, and community groups work together to support learning, children tend to do better in school, stay in school longer, and like school more.*[1(p7)]

Thus, it is not surprising that in 1997, and again in 2004, parental involvement became an integral part of IDEA. Congress found that:

> *... over 20 years of research and experience has demonstrated that the education of children with disabilities can be made more effective by ... strengthening the role of parents and ensuring that families of such children have meaningful opportunities to participate in the education of their children at school and at home.*

Who is considered to be the parent?

The term "parent" represents the person with whom the child lives and/or is legally responsible for the child's welfare. A parent could be a birth or adoptive parent, a guardian, a foster parent, or, in some cases, a surrogate parent (Sec. 300.30[a]).

How can service providers strengthen the role of the parents?

Ensuring parent involvement can be difficult, especially for physical therapists working in settings other than a family's home. There has been much discussion and controversy about exactly what constitutes parental involvement and how to strengthen the role of the parents in early intervention or school-based practices.

Defining parental involvement is complicated, largely due to situational complexities (eg, employment, number of sibling, access to resources, socioeconomic status) and cultural variables (eg, family values, beliefs, and practices). "Evidence shows that parents and educators define *involvement* differently; parents take a more community-centric view that includes keeping their children safe and getting them to school, whereas teachers define involvement primarily as parental presence at school."[2(p311)]

Table 2-1. Principles and Indicators of Collaborative Partnerships

Principle of partnership	Indicators of professional behavior
Trust	Being reliable, being discrete, using sound judgment, maintaining confidentiality, trusting yourself.
Communication	Sharing resources, clarity, honesty, communicating positively, tactfulness, openness, listening, frequent communication, coordinating information, friendliness.
Commitment	Being flexible, regarding work as more than a job, regarding the child/family as more than a case, being encouraging and consist, going above and beyond.
Professional competence/skills	Taking action, having expectations, meeting individual needs, willingness to learn, setting high expectations.
Respect	Valuing the child, being nonjudgmental and courteous, nondiscrimination, avoiding intrusion, affirming strengths, treating families and child with dignity.
Equality/advocacy	Empowering, validating, advocating for child or family with others, allowing reciprocity, being willing to explore options, fostering harmony, acting equal, preventing problems, pinpointing and documenting problems.

Because of these differences, judgments about parental involvement from school or early intervention personnel are easily and readily made. Parents may be very involved in the everyday decisions facing their families; however, some of their involvement may not be evident to early intervention or school personnel. Jackson and Remillard[3] suggested this may be the case for families with low socioeconomic status, whose parenting efforts may primarily be focused at home or work and not at school. Families, for example, may need to focus their time and energy on maintaining employment, and taking time off of work to be involved at school may be a hardship for the family. Some service providers, however, may perceive the parent as being uninvolved. Other circumstances may prevent parents from being readily available, such as an ill family member or personal health problems. If a physical therapist were to assume that parents were uninvolved without exploring the reason behind their apparent lack of involvement, the relationship between the physical therapist and parents may suffer.

Another factor influencing a parent's involvement in the school setting is a parent's sense of success within their own education and their level of competence.[4] If parents had a negative experience in their schooling, it may influence their comfort and confidence in interacting with school staff, including physical therapists.

What can service providers do to understand and support parent involvement?

A place to start is to understand how parents view themselves as involved in their child's early intervention or school experience. Understanding the way they view their involvement can provide personnel with an understanding the gap between the desired level of involvement and the current situation. When physical therapists understand this gap, strategies for supporting family involvement and opening doors for collaboration can be developed. One family, for example, may view their involvement as daily presence at the setting, whereas another family may view their involvement as monthly contact over the phone. Additional suggestions for supporting parent involvement are provided in Table 2-1.

What is a collaborative partnership?

The goal of parent involvement should be a collaborative partnership in which each person shapes the processes for information sharing to successfully occur. "Partnership" is defined as a relationship between individuals or groups that is characterized by mutual cooperation and responsibility, as for the achievement of a specified goal.[5] Collaboration, a process used to reach goals that cannot be achieved by acting alone, requires the participants to (1) jointly develop and agree to a set of common goals and directions, (2) share

Table 2-2. Tips for Parent–Professional Communication

Tool	Purpose
E-mail	Encourage parents to communicate with you through your professional email address. This can open the door to establishing a consistent communication mode and can cut down on playing "phone tag" with parents. Some parents are much better at expressing their needs and concerns in writing. This is also a good way to have written documentation of present and past events.
Communication notebook	Having the child carry a small spiral notebook back and forth between home and school can provide daily communication between school personnel and parents. A spiral notebook is recommended to avoid losing pages and disrupting the timeline of events documented in the notebook.
Personal contact card	Have a business or contact card printed that has your name, title, phone/voice mail number and email on it. On the back side, make a statement that encourages parents to contact you anytime they have questions or concerns or need additional support.
Open house	Participate in your school's open house night for parents. Send a note home to let parents know you will be available for short meetings during this event. Most schools have an open house night during the first 9 weeks of school each year.
Child portfolio	Ask parents to provide a portfolio about their child. A portfolio can include information about the child's likes/dislikes, hobbies outside of school, family photos, family tree, and anything else the family thinks is important for you to know. Portfolios are a great way to learn about children's strengths and get to know them on a more personal level. A portfolio can be a handwritten one-page document or a decorative scrapbook.

responsibility for obtaining those goals, and (3) work together to achieve those goals, using the expertise of each collaborator. When the process is enacted, the outcome will result in cohesive practices and include a shared vision of the process and goal.[6] The principle of collaborative partnerships between parents and early intervention and school personnel is core to IDEA.

What are the factors associated with an effective collaborative partnership?

Turnbull et al[7] identified 7 core principles of effective partnerships: communication, commitment, professional competence, respect, equality, advocacy, and trust. Trust has been identified as the cornerstone of these principles, because without trust a partnership may cease to exist. Much of what contributes to an effective collaborative partnership is how we as providers interact with parents.

What are professional behaviors that promote effective collaborative partnerships?

Blue-Banning et al[8] and Turnbull et al[7] described indicators of professional behavior that facilitate a collaborative partnership, which are outlined in Table 2-1.

What are some tips for effective collaboration with families in early intervention (Part C)?

In early intervention, the term "family-centered" represents a collaborative partnership between provider and parent. Family-centered early intervention emphasizes practices that capitalize on family strengths and promote family choice and control during decision making and the process of collaboration.[9] If services are provided in a family-centered manner, parents, as collaborative partners, should gain skills to enhance the

Table 2-3. Parental Activities and Roles

Activity	Role	IDEA Regulations
Input during evaluation	Consent for initial evaluation. Provide information about their child during their child's evaluation Be part of the group reviewing existing evaluation data during any evaluation or reevaluation of their child.	Sec. 300.300(a) Sec. 300.301(b) Sec. 300.301(c)(1)(i) Sec. 300.300(d)(4)(i)
Eligibility	Entitled to be part of the group that makes the decision regarding their child's eligibility.	Sec. 300.306(c)
Placement	Entitled to be part of the group that makes the decision regarding their child's educational placement. Consent for placement.	Sec. 300.116(a) Sec. 300.501(c) During pending due process: Sec. 300.504(c)(7)
Services	Consent for services.	Sec. 300.300(b) Sec. 300.300(a)(ii)
IEP	Consent to excuse IEP team members from an IEP meeting, in whole or in part, when the meeting involves a modification to or discussion of the member's area of the curriculum or related services. The parent is required to provide informed consent before a comprehensive multi-year IEP is developed.	Sec. 300.321(e)(2)(i)
Reevaluation	Provide consent for their child to be reevaluated. Participation in all meetings: Given the opportunity to participate in meetings related to the identification, evaluation, and educational placement of their child, and the provision of FAPE to their child.	Sec. 300.300(c) Sec. 300.300(c)(1)(i)

development of their child. Parents should be afforded opportunities for family involvement and leadership by serving on state and local interagency planning councils and task forces, serving as staff to state agencies and local programs, acting as trainers, and providing support, networking, and advocacy opportunities for other families. Information on parent leadership initiatives and opportunities is usually available from each state's early intervention program. Family supports and networking resources promote the vision of "families helping families" and are available from many parent centers across the country.

What are some tips for collaboration between families and physical therapists providing services under Part B?

Parents can be partners with school personnel by helping them to understand their child, participating on the IEP team, working with the IEP team to design and implement appropriate evaluation and services, and becoming meaningfully involved in the school community. Consistent open communication between parents and school personnel is the key to successful collaboration. Take time to get to know parents on a more personal level and communicate frequently with them rather than just at the annual IEP meeting. Table 2-2 provides some ways that help to achieve quality communication with the parents.

How do we know if we are effectively involving parents?

Despite the importance of parental involvement, the tools used to measure parent involvement are sparse. Most of the program evaluation tools investigate how satisfied parents are with programming. Measurement of satisfaction, however, is limited because it only provides information about whether parents liked and appreciated the services received, but not the extent to which they were involved or the benefits of this involvement. Currently, we are not aware of any tools other than satisfaction surveys. As previously suggested, service providers can certainly ask parents guided questions about how beneficial services are in promoting their involvement in the early intervention and educational programs of their children.

What is the role of the parent in the special education process?

Parents can and should assume various roles throughout the special education process. These roles are outlined according to activity and the related IDEA regulation described in Table 2-3.

What does "informed consent" mean?

"Informed consent" means that a parent has been provided with all the relevant material and information related to the reason consent is sought. For successful information sharing to occur, the request for consent must be written in the parent's native language, or another mode of communication must be obtained. If a parent is blind or has no written language the communication of the consent would need to be in Braille or the parent's other preferred form of communication. Consent is secured when a parent communicates an understanding of why the consent is sought and then signs a written consent form.

As part of the consent, the parent must create a list of people to whom the records can be released. Providing consent is a voluntary action on the part of the parent, and the parent has a right to revoke consent at any time (Sec. 300.9[c][2]).

Do parents need to consent to everything or is parental consent not required in some situations?

Although limited in number, certain circumstances do exist when parental consent is not required. If all children in the school setting, for example, are in the process of being evaluated and consent for evaluation was not necessary for these students, then consent is not needed for the child receiving special education and related services. In addition, when a physical therapist is reviewing notes and data as part of an evaluation or reevaluation, consent is not necessary (Sec. 300.300[d][1]). Just because a parent consents for evaluation, however, it should not be assumed that the parents consent for their child to receive special education and related services.

What are the steps to ensure one or both parents are present at each IEP team meeting?

Parents must be afforded the opportunity to participate, and this includes notifying parents of the meeting early enough to ensure that they will have an opportunity to attend, and scheduling the meeting at a mutually agreed on time and place (Sec. 300.322[a][2]). Even though IDEA does not specify that parents can invite other people to the meeting, it is permissible. Parents often bring an advocate or grandparent to participate in the meeting.

When must the school ensure participation from parents?

Notice must be given to the parents at the time of identification, evaluation, and placement decisions. The parents must be given an opportunity to participate in these meetings.

Does a parent have to physically attend the meeting to participate?

A parent does not have to physically attend a meeting to participate. If neither parent can attend an IEP team meeting, however, the school must use other methods to ensure parent participation, which may include individual or conference telephone calls.

May district personnel ever meet to discuss a child and not invite a parent to attend?

Parents would not need to be invited to join informal conversations such as those which occur when 2 coworkers pass in the hall and discuss intervention or the coordination of services. Another example is when therapists and other school personnel engage in discussions to develop a proposal or response to a parent's proposal that will be discussed at a later meeting. No formal decisions, however, can be made without the parent (Sec. 300.501[b]).

What if a parent refuses to participate in an IEP meeting?

If parents refuses to participate in an IEP meeting or the school is unable to obtain parents' participation in a decision, all attempts to ensure their involvement must be documented and recorded. The records should include when telephone calls were made and the results of those calls, copies of written correspondences sent to the parents, and records of attempts to visit the parent's home or place of employment and the results of these visits (Sec. 300.322[d]).

What if a parent disagrees with the findings of an evaluation?

Parents can disagree with the findings of evaluations and they have a right to another evaluation at the school's expense. The school must, without unnecessary delay, either file a due process complaint to request a hearing to show that its evaluation is appropriate or ensure that an independent educational evaluation is provided at public expense. The school can set the criteria for the independent evaluation, which can include where the evaluation takes place and the qualifications of the examiner.

If the school files for due process complaint and the original evaluation is found to be appropriate, the parent still has the right to another independent educational evaluation, but not at the school's expense. A parent is entitled to only one independent educational evaluation at public expense each time the school conducts an evaluation with which the parent disagrees (Sec. 300.502[b]).

What if the parent disagrees with the IEP?

Although disagreement with the specifics of an IEP can be expected, more often than not resolution occurs. Sometimes, however, parties are not able to negotiate to resolve the conflicts. In this case, the parties can attempt to resolve the conflict using other avenues. Under Sec. 300.153, a parent has the right to file a signed written complaint under the procedures described in Sec. 300.151 through 300.152. The complaint must include a statement regarding how the school violated a requirement of Part B, the facts on which the statement is based, the signature and contact information for the complainant, and a proposed resolution for the problem.

Parents also have the right to mediation. Mediation is a dispute resolution process that uses a trained person to assist other people in coming to a decision about how to resolve their conflict. The mediator does not decide the outcome of the dispute. The mediation process is a voluntary action on the part of both parties. Mediation should not be used to deny or delay the parent's right to due process procedures.

The final step in the conflict resolution process is an impartial due process hearing. In general, whenever a complaint has been received, the parents or the school involved in the complaint shall have an opportunity for an impartial due process hearing. The party requesting the due process is not allowed to raise issues at the due process hearing that were not raised in the notice filed, unless the other party agrees. The request for an impartial due process hearing must be filed within 2 years from the complaint. The timeline shall not apply, however, to a parent if the parent was prevented from requesting the hearing due to specific misrepresentations by the school.

What is a parent's right to review or examine their child's records?

The parents of a child with a disability must be afforded with the opportunity to inspect and review all education records (Sec. 300.613).

How does parental involvement differ under Part C of the IDEA?

Both Part B and Part C emphasize informed consent, parental participation in decision making, and ability to access records. Part C, however, includes the assessment of family resources, priorities, and concerns, as well as procedures to address the needs of the child and family. Chapter 5 will address this topic in more detail.

SUMMARY

This chapter covered expectations for parental involvement under IDEA. It introduced some ways to conceptualize parental involvement and ways to ensure effective and meaningful parental involvement. Physical therapists and others team members can make deliberate attempts to understand parents' views of their involvement, and find strategies to support parent–professional collaboration. Optimal parent–professional collaboration positively influences developmental and educational outcomes for children.

REFERENCES

1. Henderson A, Mapp K. *A New Wave of Evidence: The Impact of School, Family, and Community Connections on Student Achievement.* Austin, TX: Southwest Educational Development Laboratory, National Center for Family & Community Connections With Schools; 2002.
2. Anderson KJ, Minke KM. Parent involvement in education: toward an understanding of parents' decision making. *J Educ Res.* 2007;100:311-323.
3. Jackson K, Remillard J. Rethinking parent involvement: African American mothers construct their roles in the mathematics education of their children. *The School Community Journal.* 2005;15(1):51-73.
4. Carlisle E, Stanley L, Kemple KM. Opening doors: understanding school and family influences on family involvement. *Early Child Educ J.* 2005;33:155-162.
5. *The American Heritage Dictionary of the English Language.* 4th ed. Boston, MA: Houghton Mifflin; 2007.
6. Bruner J. The cognitive revolution in children's understanding of mind. *Hum Dev.* 1995;38:203-213.
7. Turnbull A, Turnbull R, Erwin E, Soodak L. *Families, Professional, and Exceptity: Positive Outcomes Through Partnerships and Trust.* 5th ed. Saddle River, NJ: Pearson Prentice Hall; 2006.
8. Blue-Banning M, Summers JA, Frankland HC, Nelson LL, Beegle G. Dimensions of family and professional partnerships: constructive guidelines for collaboration. *Except Child.* 2004;70:167-184.
9. Bruder MB. Family-centered early intervention: clarifying our values for the new millennium. *Top Early Child Special Educ.* 2000;20(2):105-115.

3
Deciding Who Should Receive Physical Therapy Services Under IDEA

Irene McEwen, PT, PhD, FAPTA

The process for deciding which children should receive physical therapy services has been one of the most controversial and poorly understood aspects of IDEA. This is especially true for provision of school-based physical therapy for children served under Part B. Because decisions about physical therapy as a related service are more complex than decisions about physical therapy as an early intervention service, and because some early intervention decisions are more easily understood if one has a background in school-based decisions, this chapter first covers decision-making for services under Part B.

MAKING DECISIONS ABOUT SCHOOL-BASED PHYSICAL THERAPY (PART B)

How does a team decide if a student is eligible for physical therapy in school?

The difference between "eligibility" for school-based physical therapy and "need" for school-based physical therapy is important to understand. All students who are eligible for special education and some students with disabilities who do not receive special education are eligible for physical therapy. Generally, if a student has a disability, the student can receive school-based therapy if the student's educational team decides that the student needs therapy services.

Who is eligible for special education?

Under IDEA, students are eligible for special education and related services (such as physical therapy) if they are within the age range specified by the state's plan for special education (usually ages 3 through 21), meet the eligibility criteria for one of the 13 categories of disabilities specified in IDEA or the criteria for developmental delay, and require special education and related services because of the disability (Sec. 300.8[a]).

What are the 13 categories of disabilities?

The 13 categories are autism, deaf-blindness, deafness, hearing impairment, mental retardation, multiple disabilities, orthopedic impairments, other health impairment, serious emotional disturbance, specific learning disability, speech or language impairment, traumatic brain injury, and visual impairment including blindness (Sec. 300.8[c]). For children aged 3 through 9 years, or for a subset of children within that age range, states

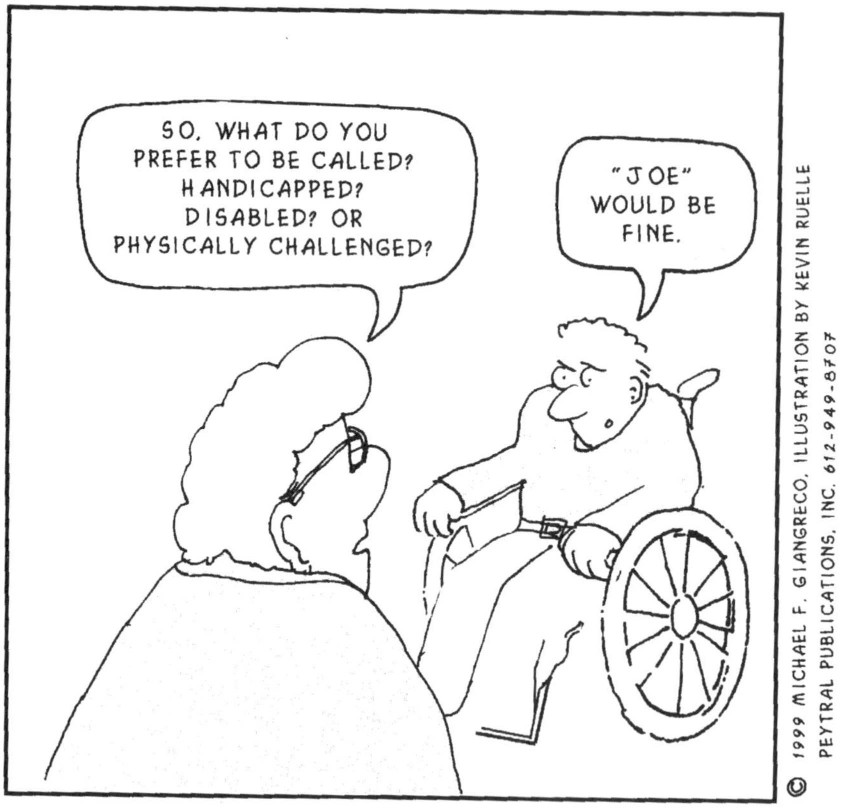
SO, WHAT DO YOU PREFER TO BE CALLED? HANDICAPPED? DISABLED? OR PHYSICALLY CHALLENGED?
"JOE" WOULD BE FINE.
© 1999 MICHAEL F. GIANGRECO, ILLUSTRATION BY KEVIN RUELLE
PEYTRAL PUBLICATIONS, INC. 612-949-8707

THE MOST APPROPRIATE LABEL IS USUALLY THE ONE PEOPLE'S PARENTS HAVE GIVEN THEM.

and local education agencies (LEAs) may choose to use the category of developmental delay, rather than label a child with a particular disability. The developmental delay category requires that children have delay in 1 or more of the following areas: physical development, cognitive development, communication development, social or emotional development, or adaptive development, and therefore need special education and related services (Sec. 300.8[b]). For more information about state and LEA requirements if they choose to use the developmental delay category, see Sec. 300.111(b).

What about children with attention deficit disorder?

The IDEA 2004 regulations address children with attention deficit disorder and attention deficit hyperactivity disorder under the category of other health impairment. The definition of other health impairment includes:

> *… a heightened alertness to environmental stimuli, that results in limited alertness with respect to the educational environment, that is due to chronic or acute health problems such as...attention deficit disorder or attention deficit hyperactivity disorder...and adversely affects a child's educational performance. (Sec. 300.8[c][9])*

Do all children with 1 or more of the disabilities (or developmental delay) qualify for special education and related services under IDEA?

No. If students' disabilities do not adversely affect their educational performance, they do not require special education and related services and do not qualify for these services under IDEA. If a child needs only a related service, not special education, the child is not considered a child with a disability under IDEA (Sec. 300.8[a][2][i]).

Under some state standards, however, physical therapy and other services that often are considered to be related services can be special education, so in those states a child needing the related service could be considered a child with a disability under IDEA and receive physical therapy as special education (Sec. 300.8[a][2][ii]). Other students whose disabilities do not adversely affect their educational performance may qualify for services and civil rights protections under Section 504 of the Rehabilitation Act of 1973 and the Americans With Disabilities Act.

Can physical therapists assist other students?

A new part of IDEA as amended in 2004 relates to "early intervening services" (not to be confused with early intervention services), which permits school districts to use not more than 15 percent of IDEA funds to:

> *... develop and implement coordinated, early intervening services, which may include interagency financing structures, for students in kindergarten through grade 12 (with a particular emphasis on students in kindergarten through grade three) who are not currently identified as needing special education or related services, but who need additional academic and behavioral support to succeed in a general education environment. (Sec. 300.226[a])*

Early intervening activities may include:

> *(1) Professional development (which may be provided by entities other than LEAs) for teachers and other school staff to enable such personnel to deliver scientifically based academic and behavioral interventions, including scientifically based literacy instruction, and, where appropriate, instruction on the use of adaptive and instructional software; and*
>
> *(2) Providing educational and behavioral evaluations, services, and supports, including scientifically based literacy instruction. (Sec. 300.226[b])*

School districts are developing processes for providing early intervening services, which could involve physical therapy for some students.

What was that about related services being special education for some students?

Physical therapy can be special education, rather than a related service, if it meets the definition of special education and can be considered special education under state standards (Sec. 300.8[a][2][ii]). Some, but not all, states permit this. Physical therapy is most often special education when students with disabilities are not receiving special education for classroom purposes. A child with spina bifida, for example, who is doing well in a general education classroom may have some other educational needs, such as self care and mobility, that can be met by receiving physical therapy as special education. In a state that does not permit physical therapy to be special education, this student might be served under Section 504. The state would not receive federal support for Section 504 services, but it would receive federal funds for services provided under IDEA.

What is "special education"?

Understanding the definition of special education is key to providing appropriate special education and related services under Part B of IDEA. The federal regulations give the following definition of special education:

> *Sec. 300.39 Special education*
>
> *(a)(1) Special education means specially designed instruction, at no cost to the parents, to meet the unique needs of a child with a disability, including—*
>
> *(i) Instruction conducted in the classroom, in the home, in hospitals and institutions, and in other settings: and*
>
> *(ii) Instruction in physical education.*
>
> *(2) Special education includes each of the following, if it meets the requirements of paragraph (a)(1) of this section:*
>
> *(i) Speech-language pathology services, or any other related services, if the service is considered special education rather than a related service under State standards;*
>
> *(ii) Travel training; and*
>
> *(iii) Vocational education.*

The definition of special education is worth repeating: "specially designed instruction, at no cost to the parents, to meet the unique needs of a child with a disability" (Sec. 300.39[a][1]). This definition has been applied time after time by hearing officers and judges when they decided the appropriateness of students' educational programs and the processes used to determine the programs. Each word is important.

"Specially designed" means that instruction can be anything that the student's educational team decides it should be and "to meet the unique needs" means that each child's needs must be considered individually. Educational decisions cannot be made by applying rules or criteria to all children with certain characteristics.[1,2] All children categorized as having multiple disabilities, for example, cannot receive a certain amount or type of special education and related service based on the classification. Each child's unique needs must be evaluated and considered in the educational program.

Does special education focus only on academics?

No. The purpose of IDEA is:

> *... to ensure that all children with disabilities have available to them a free appropriate public education that emphasizes special education and related services designed to meet their unique needs and prepare them for further education, employment, and independent living. (Sec. 300.1)*

Preparing children with disabilities for further education, employment, and independent living requires not only academic skills, but also attention to developmental and functional needs (Sec. 300.324[a][iv]). As discussed in more detail in Chapter 6, goals must be designed to:

> *... Meet the child's needs that result from the child's disability to enable the child to be involved in and make progress in the general curriculum; and*
>
> *Meet each of the child's other educational needs that results from the child's disability. Sec. 300.320(a)(2)(A-B)*

The other educational needs could be as diverse as learning basic self-care skills and mobility skills, to use a voice-accessed computer, to take public transportation, and to function at a job site. Special education and related services must then be designed to meet these and other unique needs of the student.

What is the definition of a "related service"?

IDEA defines a related service as a supportive service provided to assist a child with a disability to benefit from special education. Under Part B of IDEA, physical therapy is a related service. As stated in the federal regulation Sec. 300.34(a) Related Services:

> *Related services means transportation and such developmental, corrective, and other supportive services as are required to assist a child with a disability to benefit from special education, and includes speech-language pathology and audiology services, interpreting services, psychological services, physical and occupational therapy, recreation, including therapeutic recreation, early identification and assessment of disabilities in children, counseling services, including rehabilitation counseling, orientation and mobility services, and medical services for diagnostic or evaluation purposes. Related services also include school health services and school nurse services, social work services in schools, and parent counseling and training.*

IDEA 2004 added an exception to the definition of related services under Sec. 300. 34(b)(1):

> *(b) Exception; services that apply to children with surgically implanted devices, including cochlear implants.*
>
> > *(1) Related services do not include a medical device that is surgically implanted, the optimization of that device's functioning (eg, mapping), the maintenance of the device, or the replacement of that device.*

The regulations go on to say that a child with a surgically implanted device has a right to other related services the IEP team determines are necessary for a free and appropriate public education (FAPE) and that nothing:

> *(2) (i) Limits the responsibility of a public agency to appropriately monitor and maintain medical devices that are needed to maintain the health and safety of the child, including breathing, nutrition, or operation of other bodily functions, when the child is transported to and from school or is at school; or*
>
> *(iii) Prevents the routine checking of an external component of a surgically implanted device to make sure it is functioning properly, as required in Sec. 300.113(b).*

This means that even though a device, such as a cochlear implant or gastrostomy tube, may be surgically implanted, a child's school still is responsible for monitoring and maintaining the device if a child needs it school.

A related service that probably is not considered as often as it could be under Part B with its emphasis on the child rather than the child and family, as under Part C, is parent counseling and training. According to Sec. 300.34(c)(8):

> *(i) Parent counseling and training means assisting parents in understanding the special needs of their child;*
> *(ii) Providing parents with information about child development; and*
> *(iii) Helping parents to acquire the necessary skills that will allow them to support the implementation of their child's IEP or IFSP.*

The definition of related service says it assists a child to "benefit from special education." What does this mean?

Those 4 words have caused more confusion and controversy among therapists—and among teachers, parents, and physicians—than almost any other part of the law. Some people think the phrase means that related services must support a child's reading, writing, and arithmetic, or other academic work. Others think it means that related services can only help a child with access to and participation in the educational environment. Actually, as discussed above, special education can mean whatever a student's individualized education program (IEP) team decides it should be—and related services are provided if the child needs them to benefit from the program.

What does "required to assist" mean?

Court cases have helped define the phrase. Two cases dealing with related services went all the way to the US Supreme Court: *Irving Independent School District v Tatro*[3] in 1980 and *Cedar Rapids Community School District v Garret F*[4] in 1999.

In the first case, Amber Tatro had spina bifida and needed clean intermittent catheterization during the school day. The school district refused to provide assistance, saying clean intermittent catheterization was a medical procedure, which is not covered by IDEA, and that it was not necessary for her to benefit from education. After 10 years (by which time Amber could catheterize herself), the US Supreme Court heard the case. The court determined that clean intermittent catheterization is a related service if a child with a disability needs it to remain at school and have access to education. Because the service could be provided by a school nurse or qualified layperson, it was not considered a "medical service."

Similarly, in 1999, the Supreme Court ruled on a case that involved Garret Frey, a Cedar Rapids, Iowa, high school student who had a spinal cord injury in childhood. He used a power wheelchair, had a tracheotomy and ventilator, and was catheterized during the school day. His school district refused to pay for the assistance he needed during the school day, saying that he required "medical treatment" for which his family would have to pay. The Court ruled that school districts must provide health supports for students who need them to attend school, as long as they are not medical in nature and performed by doctors.

Although related services were ruled to be essential for Amber and Garret to attend school, other cases courts have found that related services only need to assist a student to benefit from special education, a less rigorous standard.[5] Related services do not need to be provided to "maximize" a student's opportunities. In *Board of Education of the Hendrick Hudson Central School District v Rowley*,[6] the US Supreme Court declared that IDEA requires school districts to provide an "appropriate" education, not the best possible education. Amy Rowley was deaf and doing better than average in general education classes with some support services. She might have done even better if she had a sign language interpreter, which her parents requested. The Supreme Court determined that Amy was benefiting from her educational program without an interpreter and that school districts only have to provide a "basic floor of opportunity" and do not have to maximize the potential of children with disabilities with opportunities commensurate with those of students without disabilities.[6] See Section II, "Court Decisions, State Education Agency Hearings, Letters of Inquiry, Policy Interpretations, and Investigations by Federal Agencies Related to School-Based Physical Therapy" on page 147 for more information.

Does IDEA say what type of physical therapy is appropriate in schools?

No. Physical therapy is defined under Part B of IDEA as "services provided by a qualified physical therapist" (Sec. 300.34[c][9]). This definition means that anything that is within the scope of physical therapist practice and that the IEP team decides is "required to assist a child with a disability to benefit from special education" is appropriate.

How does the IEP team decide if a student needs physical therapy in school?

As covered in detail in Chapter 6, the IEP team develops each student's individualized education program, based on the student's unique needs. The team then decides if a student needs physical therapy to assist with achieving the educational goals, or accessing and participating in the educational environment, including extracurricular activities (Sec. 300.117).

Can educational goals be physical therapy goals?

Educational goals are discipline-free; that is, they are the goals that a student's educational team decides are appropriate for the student, given a student's unique needs. Team members should not write separate "academic goals," "physical therapy goals," "speech goals," and so forth. IDEA does not require that goals be written for each discipline (see p. 46662 in "Analysis of Comments and Changes in 34 CFR 300" in the CD with this book) and best practices strongly support writing goals that are discipline free.[7,8]

Obviously, the unique educational needs of many students with disabilities must encompass more than academic subjects to prepare them for adulthood. If a student has motor problems, some of the student's educational goals may relate to motor skills, such as mobility or self-help skills. Depending on the expertise of other educational team members, including the student's teacher and other related services providers, physical therapy may or may not be needed to assist the student to achieve those educational goals.

Why might a student need physical therapy to assist with access to and participation in the educational environment?

Some activities that take place during the school day are not directly related to achieving goals, but are required for students to remain in the educational environment and have the opportunity to work toward their goals. These activities assist students with access to and participation in the educational environment. Some students, for example, must be fed, others must have their diapers changed, be catheterized, or transferred to a toilet. Students with severe motor impairments often need to have their position changed throughout the day or they may need some means of moving from place to place.

The services that students need other people to do for them so they can attend school are not written as goals and objectives for the student to achieve. As described in Chapter 6, they are documented on the IEP as services that are provided so the student can have access to and participate in the educational environment. A physical therapist, for example, may be needed to identify and acquire appropriate positioning devices for a child and teach classroom personnel how to use the equipment, show a paraprofessional how to transfer a student in the bathroom, or teach peers how to push the wheelchair of a student without an independent means of mobility.

Do guidelines or policies exist to help make decisions about physical therapy?

Many physical therapists, school administrators, and others have tried to develop simple and "objective" methods to decide which students are "eligible" for physical therapy in school or to decide how much and what kind of physical therapy to provide. Some districts, for example, have rules stating that students whose cognitive abilities measure lower than their motor abilities are "ineligible" for physical therapy. Others have guidelines saying students must score so many standard deviations below the mean on a test of gross motor development to "qualify" for physical therapy, or that students over a certain age, students who attend certain schools, or students who have certain diagnoses are eligible for only certain types of physical therapy services, such as consultation with teachers.

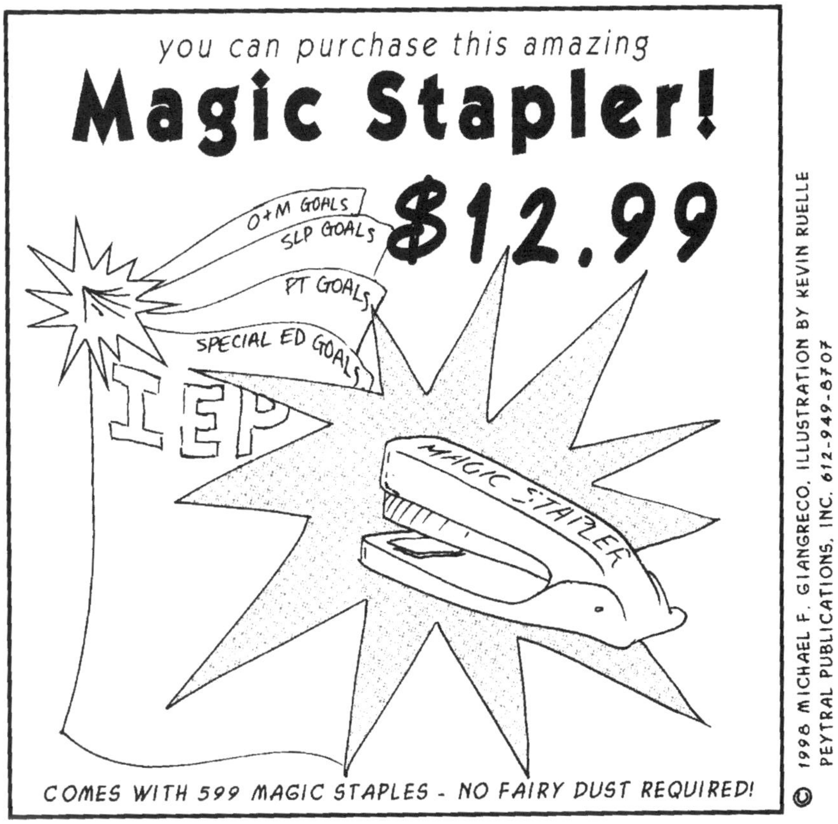
you can purchase this amazing
Magic Stapler!
$12.99
O+M GOALS
SLP GOALS
PT GOALS
SPECIAL ED GOALS
IEP
MAGIC STAPLER
COMES WITH 599 MAGIC STAPLES - NO FAIRY DUST REQUIRED!
© 1998 MICHAEL F. GIANGRECO, ILLUSTRATION BY KEVIN RUELLE
PEYTRAL PUBLICATIONS, INC. 612-949-8707

TRANSFORM YOUR SEPARATE, DISJOINTED, DISCIPLINE-SPECIFIC, UNCOORDINATED GOALS INTO A "TEAM IEP."

Based on answers to previous questions, eligibility clearly is not the issue. All students with disabilities are eligible for physical therapy. The question to ask is, "Does a student need physical therapy?" Students' educational teams have the responsibility and the authority to make this decision and, if a student needs physical therapy, to decide on the type and intensity of services to provide. The US Office of Special Education Programs (OSEP) has made it clear that any guideline or policy violates IDEA if it categorically denies services to students with certain characteristics, or limits an IEP team's ability to make decisions based on assessment of students' individual and unique needs.[1]

What is the difference between "educational" therapy and "medical" therapy?

Many pediatric physical therapists, administrators, and other school personnel have attempted to differentiate between "educational" therapy and "medical" therapy. The effort grew out of the requirement for physical therapy services provided under IDEA to relate to students' educational programs. As all pediatric therapy has become more family-centered and more oriented toward functional goals, however, and as the definition of "educational" has broadened beyond traditional academic pursuits, former differences in therapy provided for students with disabilities in clinical and educational environments have largely disappeared.[8] The difference is in the priorities, not in the type of therapy provided.

In educational environments, the team decides on the educational program for a student with a disability (see Chapter 6 for details of this process). If a team decides, for example, that learning to walk independently is a high priority for a student, given everything the physical therapist and other team members know about the student and the likelihood that the student can learn to walk, then independent ambulation would be included in the IEP. In this case, physical therapy to help the student learn to walk could be identical to physical therapy provided in a clinical setting. In either setting, the most effective methods should be used; "educational methods" are not used in one setting and "medical methods" in the other.

On the other hand, if the team (including the family and physical therapist) decides that walking is not a priority in a student's educational program, then walking would not be an educational goal and the school-based therapist would not work with the student on walking. Walking might not be selected as an educational priority because the team decides that other goals are more important or because walking is not likely to be achieved. When other educational goals take priority, the family may seek physical therapy services that are not paid by the school district to help the child learn to walk. If the child were not likely to learn to walk, however, the goal would be inappropriate regardless of the setting.

Can students with disabilities who attend private schools receive school therapy services at public expense?

When Congress amended IDEA in 1997 and 2004, it attempted to clarify parents' and LEA rights and responsibilities when students attend private schools. In general, students with disabilities who attend private schools can receive therapy services at school district expense if they have been placed in or referred to the school by a public agency as a means of providing special education and related services (Sec. 300.146).

When parents unilaterally place their child with a disability in a private school, including religious schools, then the school district in which the private school is located has certain other responsibilities. One of those responsibilities is to identify the children, evaluate them, and ensure they have equitable participation under IDEA (Sec. 300.131), including special education and related services (Sec. 300.132[a]) that are to be documented on a services plan (Sec. 300.132[b]). Sec. 300.133 gives formulae to determine how much each LEA must spend to provide special education and related services for students with disabilities whose parents place them in private schools. The regulations go on to say:

> *Sec. 300.137(a) No parentally-placed private school child with a disability has an individual right to receive some or all of the special education and related services that the child would receive if enrolled in public school.*
>
> *Sec. 300.137(c) If a child with a disability is enrolled in a religious or other private school by the child's parents and will receive special education and related services from the LEA, the LEA must –*
>
> *(1) Initiate and conduct meetings to develop, review, and revise a service plan for the child, in accordance with Sec. 300.138(b); and*
>
> *(2) Ensure that a representative of the religious or other private school attends each meeting. If the representative cannot attend, the LEA shall use other methods to ensure participation by the religious or other private schools, including individual or conference telephone calls.*

Children whose parents place them in private schools do not need to receive the same amount of services that children with disabilities in public schools receive (Sec. 300.138[a][2]). Services may be provided on site at the private school, including religious schools, or the child may be provided transportation, if necessary, to benefit from and participate in services (Sec. 300.139[a-b]). Public school personnel can provide services at other than public facilities (Sec. 300.142), although off-site physical therapy services should be avoided whenever possible because proximity to the child's school environment is important if physical therapy is to support the child's educational program. Motor learning, for example, is enhanced by practice in the environments in which the skill will be used, and opportunities for consultation with school personnel are much more likely when the child is seen at school than when transported to another location.

In some cases, parents who place their child with a disability in a private school at their own expense or who home school the child may not consent to evaluation or want special education and related services. A new section in IDEA 2004 clarifies that parents have the option of not participating and may opt out of public school services if they choose (Sec. 300.300[d][4]).

For more information about provision of services for children in private schools including regulations related to provision of necessary equipment see Sec. 300.129-148 included in the accompanying CD. Another good resource for information on this complex topic is a book on IDEA 2004 regulations by Richards and Martin.[9]

Can students with disabilities who are home-schooled receive physical therapy services at public expense?

The answer to this question depends on State law. According to the Analysis of Comments and Changes section of the regulations in the accompanying CD:

> *Whether home-schooled children with disabilities are considered parentally-placed private school children with disabilities is a matter left to State law. Children with disabilities in home schools or home day cares must be treated in the same way as other parentally-placed private school children with disabilities for purposes of Part B of the Act only if the State recognizes home schools or home day cares as private elementary schools or secondary schools* (71 FR 46594)

MAKING DECISIONS ABOUT PHYSICAL THERAPY IN EARLY INTERVENTION PROGRAMS

How are decisions made about physical therapy for infants or toddlers under Part C?

As is the case for older children with disabilities, infants and toddlers are "eligible" for physical therapy if they qualify for services under IDEA. Once a child is determined eligible for early intervention services, the question to be answered is, does the child need physical therapy?

Who is eligible for services under Part C?

Infants, toddlers, and their families are eligible for Part C services if the children meet the definition of "infants and toddlers with disabilities."

Sec. 303.21 Infants or toddlers with a disability.

(a) Infant or toddler with a disability means an individual under three years of age who needs early intervention services because the individual—

(1) Is experiencing a developmental delay, as measured by appropriate diagnostic instruments and procedures, in one or more of the following areas:

(i) Cognitive development.

(ii) Physical development, including vision and hearing.

(iii) Communication development.

(iv) Social or emotional development.

(v) Adaptive development; or

(2) Has a diagnosed physical or mental condition that—

(i) Has a high probability of resulting in developmental delay; and

(ii) Includes conditions such as chromosomal abnormalities; genetic or congenital disorders; severe sensory impairments; inborn errors of metabolism; disorders reflecting disturbance of the development of the nervous system; congenital infections; and disorders secondary to exposure to toxic substances, including fetal alcohol syndrome.

These regulations mean that infants and toddlers can qualify for early intervention services if they (1) are delayed in the areas of cognitive, physical (including sensory and motor), communication, social or emotional, and/or adaptive (self-help) development; or (2) have a condition that is likely to result in developmental delay, such as Down syndrome, whether or not they are delayed at the time of evaluation.

States may choose to include children at risk for disabilities (Sec. 303.21[b]). They also may choose to provide early intervention services for young children who are eligible for Part B preschool services until they enter or are eligible to enter kindergarten or elementary school under state law (Sec. 303.21[c]).

Do all states have the same eligibility criteria?

No. The amount of developmental delay, the specific conditions, and the type of risk that qualifies a child for early intervention services are left to the states' discretion, within federal guidelines (Sec. 303.111)

Because each state has its own eligibility criteria and procedures, it is important for physical therapists providing services under Part C to obtain and review these criteria for their own states. Chapter 4, "Evaluation and Assessment," covers general information about evaluation to determine eligibility for Part C services.

Is physical therapy a "related service" under Part C, as it is under Part B?

No. Under Part C, physical therapy is an "early intervention service."

What is an early intervention service?

The general definition of early intervention services is:

> *Sec. 303.13 Early intervention services.*
>
> *(a) General. Early intervention services means developmental services that—*
>
> *(1) Are provided under public supervision;*
> *(2) Are selected in collaboration with the parents;*
> *(3) Are provided at no cost, except, subject to Sec. 303.520 and 303.521, where Federal or State law provides for a system of payments by families, including a schedule of sliding fees;*
> *(4) Are designed to meet the developmental needs of an infant or toddler with a disability and as requested by the family, the needs of the family to assist appropriately in the infant's or toddler's development, as identified by the individualized family service plan team, in any one or more of the following areas, including—*
> *(i) Physical development;*
> *(ii) Cognitive development;*
> *(iii) Communication development;*
> *(iv) Social or emotional development; or*
> *(v) Adaptive development;*
> *(5) Meet the standards of the State in which the services are provided, including the requirements of Part C of the Act;*
> *(6) Include services identified under paragraph (b) of this section;*
> *(7) Are provided by qualified personnel (as that term is defined in Sec. 303.31), including the types of personnel listed in paragraph (c) of this section;*
> *(8) To the maximum extent appropriate, are provided in natural environments, as defined in Sec. 303.26 and consistent with Sec. 303.126; and*
> *(9) Are provided in conformity with an individualized family service plan adopted in accordance with section 636 of the Act and Sec. 303.20.*

What are the services "identified under paragraph (b) of this section"?

Fourteen early intervention services are listed and defined under Sec. 303.13(b). They include assistive technology, audiology, family training, health services, medical services only for diagnostic or evaluation purposes, occupational therapy, physical therapy, psychological services, service coordination services, social work services, special instruction, speech-language pathology services, transportation and related costs, and vision services.

Are these the only services that states can provide?

No. Sec. 303.13(d) clearly states that the list is not exhaustive. It says:

> *The services and personnel identified and defined in paragraphs (b) and (c) of this section do not comprise exhaustive lists of the types of services that may constitute early intervention services or the types of qualified personnel that may provide early intervention services. Nothing in this section prohibits the identification on the IFSP of another type of service as an early intervention service provided that the service meets the criteria identified in paragraph (a) of this section or of another type of personnel that may provide early intervention services in accordance with this part, provided such personnel meet the requirements in Sec. 303.31.*

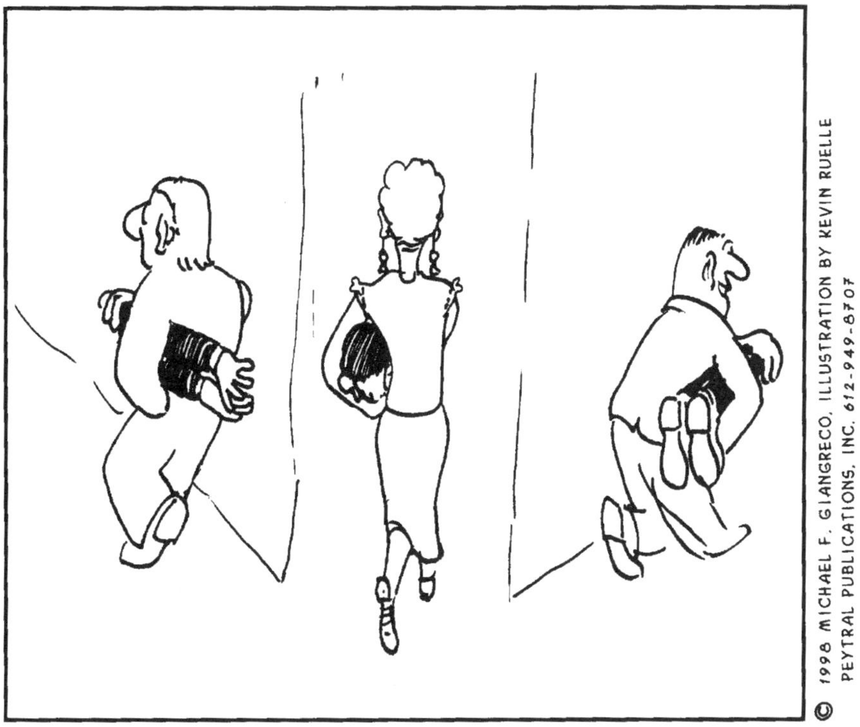

SEVERELY DYSFUNCTIONAL TEAM

What does "qualified personnel" mean in the definition of early intervention service?

Sec. 303.31 defines the term as:

> *Qualified personnel means personnel who have met State approved or recognized certification, licensing, registration, or other comparable requirements that apply to the area in which the individuals are providing early intervention services.*

Is the definition of "physical therapy" different in Part C than in Part B?

Yes. "Physical therapy" is defined more thoroughly in Part C than in Part B. Sec. 303.13(a)(7) says:

> *Physical therapy includes services to address the promotion of sensorimotor function through enhancement of musculoskeletal status, neurobehavioral organization, perceptual and motor development, cardiopulmonary status, and effective environmental adaptation. These services include—*
> *(i) Screening, evaluation, and assessment of children to identify movement dysfunction;*
> *(ii) Obtaining, interpreting, and integrating information appropriate to program planning to prevent, alleviate, or compensate for movement dysfunction and related functional problems; and*
> *(iii) Providing individual and group services or treatment to prevent, alleviate, or compensate for, movement dysfunction and related functional problems.*

How are decisions made about whether a child needs physical therapy as an early intervention service?

Just as students' educational teams make decisions about students' needs for physical therapy as a related service in school, early intervention teams make decisions about infants' and toddlers' needs for physical therapy. When the team, including the parents, meets to develop the IFSP, team members decide which services the child and family need. See Chapter 5, "Individualized Family Service Plans," for information about the IFSP process.

SUMMARY

Deciding which children should receive physical therapy as an early intervention or related service often has been controversial, particularly deciding when to provide physical therapy as a related service under Part B. Under IDEA, no "eligibility" criteria exist, however, for physical therapy services other than a child's being eligible for Part B or Part C services and the team's decision that the child needs physical therapy. The ways in which the teams make the decision are described in Chapters 5 and 6.

REFERENCES

1. Letter to Rainforth, 17 Education for the Handicapped Law Reporter (EHLR) 222 (1990).
2. Rainforth B. OSERS clarifies legality of related services eligibility criteria. *TASH Newsletter.* 1991:April:8.
3. *Irving Independent School District v Tatro,* 468 US 883 (1984).
4. *Cedar Rapids Community School District v Garret F,* 525 US 66 (1999).
5. *Norton Public School District,* 21 IDELR 974 (SEA Vt 1994).
6. *Board of Education of the Hendrick Hudson Central School District v Rowley,* 458 US 176 (1982).
7. Giangreco MF, Cloninger CJ, Iverson VS. *Choosing Outcomes and Accommodations for Children (COACH): A Guide to Educational Planning for Students With Disabilities.* 2nd ed. Baltimore, MD: Paul H. Brookes; 1998.
8. McEwen IR, Shelden ML. Pediatric physical therapy in the 1990s: the demise of the educational versus medical dichotomy. *Phys Occup Ther Pediatr.* 1995;15(2):33-45.
9. Richards DM, Martin JL. *2006 IDEA Final Part B Regulations: What You Need to Know.* Horsham, PA: LRP Publications; 2006.

4
Evaluation and Assessment

Thubi H A Kolobe, PT, PhD

Physical therapists who work with children and families participating in programs regulated by Part C and Part B of the Individuals With Disabilities Education Act, as amended by the Individuals With Disabilities Education Improvement Act of 2004 (IDEA, 2004) are expected to conduct comprehensive assessments and evaluations. The process of assessment and evaluation requires not only gathering information using a variety of tools and approaches, but also using the information to make decisions about children's eligibility for Part C or Part B services, guide the development of the goals, determine types of interventions, and evaluate whether the goals of interventions have been achieved. Consequently, it is important to understand the criteria for selecting any information-gathering method, approach, or tool, given that interpretations of such information have far-reaching consequences for the children and their families. This chapter will discuss assessment and evaluation as stipulated in Part C and Part B, with emphasis on a quantitative approach to gathering information.

How does Part C define "assessment"?

Sec. 303.320 defines assessment under 3 areas: child, family, and service needs.

Assessment of the child:

> *… means reviewing available pertinent records that relate to the child's current health status and medical history and conducting personal observation and assessment of the child in order to identify the child's unique strengths and needs, including an identification of the child's level of functioning in each of the following developmental areas: cognitive development; physical development, including vision and hearing; communication development; social or emotional development; and adaptive development. Qualified personnel must use their informed clinical opinion to assess a child's present level of functioning in each of the developmental areas identified in Sec. 303.21(a)(1).*

Assessment of the family:

> *… means identification of the family's resources, priorities, and concerns, and the supports and services necessary to enhance the family's capacity to meet the developmental needs of the family's infant or toddler with a disability, as determined not just through the use of an assessment tool, but through a voluntary personal interview with the family.*

Assessment of service needs:

> *... If the child meets the definition of infant or toddler with a disability in Sec. 303.21, an assessment of the service needs of the infant or toddler with a disability and the child's family must include a review of the evaluation (including the assessment of the child and family) and available pertinent records and conducting personal observation and assessment of the infant or toddler with a disability in order to identify the early intervention services appropriate to meet the child's unique needs in each of the developmental areas identified in paragraph (b)(1) of this section.*

These provisions imply that the assessment process for the child must include identification of the child's strengths and needs and level of functioning within different developmental domains. The process is intended to provide a picture of the child's abilities and needs for eligibility purposes as well as service planning, provided the child is eligible for Part C services. Physical therapists, as "qualified personnel" (Sec. 303.13[c][7]), can also use informed clinical opinion to establish a child's eligibility even if instruments that are designed to identify children with developmental delays (such as the Peabody Developmental Motor Scales, 2nd ed,[1] (PDMS II) or the Battelle Developmental Inventory, 2nd ed,[2] (BDI II) do not support eligibility. Sec. 303.320(b)(2) further states that "qualified personnel" (see page 47 for a definition) must use their informed clinical opinion to evaluate a child's present level of functioning in each developmental areas and that the lead agency must ensure that informed clinical opinion may be used by qualified personnel. A physical therapist cannot use the clinical informed opinion, however, to negate findings that suggest that the child has delays based on an assessment tool.

The use of informed clinical opinion suggests that assessment procedures for children with delays in the motor domain should involve personnel who are familiar with personal and environmental factors, such as brain insult, that may indicate underlying constraints to motor development or performance. Personnel with knowledge of movement and its constraints must also be part of the multidisciplinary evaluation team, particularly if the child demonstrates developmental delays associated with mobility.

Assessment of the family is voluntary; focuses on the family's resources, priorities, and concerns; and should not solely be based an assessment tool, but also on a voluntary personal interview with the family. Assessment of service needs is supposed to be completed following eligibility determination. Team members are supposed to use all available information in addition to observation and additional assessments as needed to identify the early intervention services required to meet the child's unique needs. According to Part C, assessment of service needs must involve assessment information about the child's functional status and assessment of the family's resources and needs, essentially requiring integration of the interpretation of findings from assessment results, predictions about outcome (prognosis), and analysis of existing resources.

How does Part C define "evaluation"?

> *As used in Sec. 303.322(i) an evaluation is the method used to review the assessments of the child and the family to determine a child's initial and continuing eligibility under this part, consistent with the definition of infant or toddler with a disability in Sec. 303.21.*
>
> *(ii) In conducting an evaluation, no single procedure may be used as the sole criterion for determining a child's eligibility under this part.*
>
> *(iii) A child's medical and other records may be used to establish eligibility (without conducting an assessment of the child and the family) if those records contain information required under this section regarding the child's level of functioning in the developmental areas identified in Sec. 303.21(a)(1).*

Based on this definition, physical therapists and other team members "evaluate" infants and toddlers to determine if they meet the state's eligibility criteria for early intervention services (see Chapter 3 for Part C eligibility criteria). When conducting such evaluations, no single procedure can be used to determine a child's eligibility. Procedures many include family interviews, clinical observations, and developmental tests. Medical records that contain information about the child's developmental status can be used to establish eligibility without additional testing. This may be particularly true for children who are discharged from neonatal intensive care units (NICUs) that use neonatal screening and medical diagnostic tools as part of developmental care. Such evaluations must also include assessment of the child's unique strengths and needs and identification of the child's level of functioning within the different developmental domains (social-emotional, physical, communication, adaptive, and cognitive).

IDEA 2004 Part C regulations have attempted to clarify the distinction between "evaluation" and "assessment." In short, evaluation can be thought of as an appraisal and interpretation of assessment information. An example is a 13-month-old infant who obtains a score of -1.5 standard deviation (SD) on the Peabody Developmental Motor Scale (PDMS-II).[1] Suppose a state's cut-off for eligibility is a standard deviation of -2. If the infant was also born at 30 weeks gestational age, has a neonatal history of many medical complications, and is described by the caregiver as feeding poorly, the physical therapists can use this information, with the results of the PDMS II, to determine whether or not the child has or is at risk for developmental delays.

How do physical therapists help evaluate an infant or toddler to determine eligibility for Part C services?

To determine whether or not a child has developmental delays, the child's performance is often compared with that of other children the same age through the use of norm-referenced tests. Sometimes children can be compared against an established criterion using criterion-referenced tests. Many state policies and procedures require norm-referenced tests with a specified cut-off score to determine eligibility. A few will accept a criterion-referenced test. Physical therapists use a variety of norm- and criterion-referenced tools to determine whether or not child has developmental delays, particularly motor delay.

Physical therapists need to understand the advantages and disadvantages of using test scores and the various cut-off points to determine whether or not a child has delays. Cut-off scores and judgment go hand in hand. The premise is that no matter where one draws the line, a certain amount of error in classification is to be expected (sensitivity and specificity). The decision about the cut-off score is a balancing act of how much error one is willing to live with.[2] In other words, every decision that is based on tests and measures (norm- or criterion referenced), as well as observations and interviews, have a certain amount of error associated with it. The use of confidence intervals or standard error of measurement when interpreting the results of test scores is valuable in this regard.

Cut-off points that are used by many states to determine eligibility, such as 25%, 30%, or 50% delays are also a concern. Andersson[3] presents a thorough discussion of the disadvantages of using developmental quotients, such as the age-equivalent scores or percent delay based on norm-referenced or criterion-reference tests to determine eligibility. For example, children can attain scores that places them in a specific age level of development, but this does not mean that they performs the same as typical children of that age. Age-equivalent scores of norm-referenced tests are based on mathematical or statistical calculations and not on the actual performance of the children used to develop the scale. Also, a change in 1 or 2 test items might disproportionately increase the child's age-equivalent score but not the standard score. Because children's development does not occur in equal segments, a specific percentage delay does not mean the same at all ages of development, particularly at the lower or higher ends of the age interval. A child who passes 10 items at the lower end has different abilities as the child who passes 10 items at the higher end.

What are other considerations when selecting and interpreting tests?

Physical therapists should also critically review the tools that are being used in their states or centers to determine eligibility and familiarize themselves with the tools' sensitivity and specificity and their positive and negative predictive values. Definitions by Fletcher et al[4] may be helpful. *Sensitivity* refers to the proportion of individuals classified as abnormal by the reference measure (or gold standard) who were classified as such by the scale being used. It answers the question: Of the children that the criterion measure identified as delayed, how many were identified as delayed by the scale one wants to use? *Specificity* refers to the proportion of individuals classified as "normal" by a criterion measure of the scale one is using. That is, of the number of the children that the criterion measure identified as not delayed, how many were identified as such by that particular scale? Both sensitivity and specificity help guide the decision on whether or not to choose a certain tool. Sensitivity scores above 70% are considered "acceptable"; specificity scores greater than 80% are considered "realistic." The specificity of more than 90% is considered acceptable.[5]

Positive predictive value refers to the proportion of individuals identified by the cut-off score or point as being abnormal who are classified as having a target condition by a criterion measure. It answers the question: Of the children who are identified by the tool as having delays, how many did indeed have delays? Negative predictive value refers to the proportion of individuals identified by the cut-off score or point as being normal who are classified as not having a target condition by a criterion measure. These values are concerned with *interpretation* of the test results. They help answer the question: Given the results of the test, what is the probability that the child tested does or does not have developmental delay or disability? The positive and negative predictive values focus on what the scores mean once the tool has been selected; positive predictive values above 50% are considered acceptable.[5]

Although criterion-referenced tests may be used to determine eligibility, not all yield information with cut-off points. For example, the Gross Motor Function Measure (GMFM)[6] is a criterion-referenced measure, but it can not be used as a criterion for diagnosis because the scores cannot be used to determine whether or not the child is delayed. The Pediatric Evaluation of Disability Inventory (PEDI),[7] on the other hand, is a criterion-referenced and a norm-referenced measure. The scaled score represents the criterion-referenced characteristic, and the standard scores the norm-reference attribute. However, the scaled score of the PEDI cannot be used to determine eligibility. Examples of tests that physical therapists can use to help determine eligibility for Part C or B services are described in the next sections.

Who can administer tests to determine eligibility?

It is important to understand that any appropriately trained person can administer tests to establish that a child has a developmental delay and is eligible for early intervention services. It is not required that a physical therapist be the one to administer a gross motor test to determine that a child has delayed gross motor development. Similarly, a physical therapist with appropriate training can administer tests that are used to determine if a child has delays in communication, cognitive development, or other non-motor domains. The purpose of this type of evaluation is simply to determine if the child has delays—not to identify the cause of the delay, the implications of the delay, or what to do about the delay. Physical therapists working in early intervention programs should obtain and read their own states' policies and procedures that describe test requirements, use of informed clinical opinion, and how delays must be documented for eligibility purposes, such as percentiles, percentages, standard deviations, or some other method.

Another way that physical therapists can contribute to determining whether or not an infant or toddler meets eligibility criteria is through informed clinical opinion. Sec. 303.320(b)(2) states:

> *... qualified personnel must use their informed clinical opinion to assess a child's present level of functioning in each of the developmental areas identified in Sec.303.21(a)(1) and the lead agency must ensure that informed clinical opinion may be used by qualified personnel to establish a child's eligibility under this part even when other instruments do not establish eligibility, but informed clinical opinion may not negate the results of assessment instruments used under paragraph (b)(1) of this section to establish eligibility.*

Clinical opinion implies that physical therapists can integrate information gathered from various sources and, based on knowledge unique to their discipline and development of children with disabilities, formulate a diagnosis. Clinical opinion involves a process of interpreting information obtained from sources such as interviews, observations, and tests. It requires formulation of working hypotheses and refining the working hypotheses to specific entities and relationships that can be observed or tested.[8-10] Mattingly and Fleming[9] described a process of clinical reasoning, conditional reasoning, that involves gathering information about the child and environment, making meaning out of the information presented, developing a working hypothesis (eg, a child's difficulty in feeding himself may be associated with sensory defensiveness, difficulty in swallowing, or need for head support), speculating on what information is needed to test the hypothesis (eg, oral-motor assessment), and refining the working hypothesis. The information from tests would help determine the extent of deficits in the areas tested.

What tools do physical therapists most often use to assess children?

Instruments that are used to determine eligibility for services may or may not be useful for planning programs or evaluating outcomes, especially when children have severe delays. Kirshner and Guyatt[11] described 3 types of measures: discriminative, predictive, and evaluative. Understanding the difference between these types of measures can help physical therapists use tools that are appropriate for the purpose.

What is a discriminative measure?

Discriminative measures are used to distinguish among individuals on some feature of interest, obtain data for diagnosis, or evaluate decisions.[11] They are useful to determine a child's eligibility for early intervention under Part C. Discriminative tools can be classified further into norm- and criterion-referenced tests. A norm-referenced test is designed to examine an individual's performance in relation to the performance of a representative group; it measures individual achievement against an external standard (norms). In norm-referenced tests standard scores are used rather than individual raw scores. Raw scores are meaningless until they are converted into standard scores such as percentile- or z-scores. Therefore, if the purpose of a test is to identify children with developmental delays or to determine their performance level relative to their peers, a norm-referenced test would be most appropriate. Examples of such tests are: the Bayley Scales of Infant Development-III (BSID-III)[12]; the Peabody Developmental Motor Scales, 2nd edition (PDMS-2)[1]; the Alberta Infant Motor Scale (AIMS)[13]; the Battelle Developmental Inventory, 2nd edition (BDI-2)[14]; and the Test of Infant Motor Performance (TIMP).[15] Some, like the BDI-2 and BSID-III, are comprehensive and examine performance in several domains such as adaptive behavior, cognition, communication, motor, and personal-social skills.

Criterion tests, on the other hand, measure a child's performance against external criteria, such as the highest score one can obtain on a given test, and scoring is based on absolute rather than relative standards, such as 76/100%. The primary use of criterion-referenced tests is to measure mastery of specific skills. The test items are based on known performance objectives, such as items on the Gross Motor Function Measure.[6] In some tests, items are clustered into a developmental age level, which in most cases are close to, if not the same as, the chronological ages of the sample who passed the items. Criterion-referenced tests are most appropriate to use with heterogeneous groups or to measure specific skills, such as balance. A criterion-referenced measure that is used to determine eligibility must provide a criterion that can be used to determine whether or not the child's performance is appropriate for age. One criterion-referenced test that physical therapists often use is the Hawaii Early Learning Profile (HELP).[16]

What is a "predictive measure"?

A *predictive measure* can help identify infants and toddlers who will have developmental delays in the future, particularly those with conditions with risk factors that put them at a high probability for delay. Infants who are born at very low gestational age and birth weight often fit into this category. When combined with informed clinical opinion, a predictive measure may be useful to determine whether a child is eligible for early intervention services. Examples of predictive tools are the TIMP and AIMS.[15,17] Screening tools in general also serve a predictive role. Examples are the Harris Infant Neuromotor Test (HINT),[18] the Test of Infant Motor Performance Screening Items (TIMPSI),[19] and Ages and Stages Questionnaires.[20] Predictive tools are limited not only to developmental tests. Other measures can be used to predict development of secondary complication or absence thereof, such as the inclinometer for scoliosis, or a goniometer for joint contractures that may require orthoses or surgery.

Some predictive measures are useful for program planning. A measure that predicts whether a young child with cerebral palsy will walk, for example, could be helpful in deciding what to emphasize in a therapy program (see Chapter 9). Predictive tests are rare because of the difficulty in accurately predicting outcome in infants and toddlers.

What is an "evaluative measure"?

Evaluative measures are used to determine change over time or change as the result of intervention. Many tests that are useful for identifying children with delays or predicting which children will have problems later on are not especially useful for assessing change over time. In addition to reliability and validity, an evaluative measure must demonstrate responsiveness. The reliability of an evaluative test should be demonstrated by stable intra-subject variation in scores between testing, and the validity by a relationship between changes in test score and an external measure over time.[11]

A question often asked is, what the difference between responsiveness and sensitivity? Responsiveness of an evaluative measure is the test's ability to detect minimal clinically important differences, when such change occurs.[21] The sensitivity of an evaluative measure, like that of a discriminative test, is its ability to accurately and appropriately identify individuals who have changed and those who did not.[11] According to Guyatt et al,[21] responsiveness of a test is directly related to the magnitude of the change in the person's score that constitutes a clinically important difference. Therefore the question that responsiveness addresses in an evaluative measure is: Has clinically important change occurred? Or has functionally important change occurred? In other words, is the change from 18 to 19 months age-equivalent score (based on the PDMS-2 or any other measure) clinically/functionally significant? Often studies that evaluate the responsiveness of a test are published after the test has been published.

Evaluative measures of change in motor outcome are rare. The GMFM is the only motor test that was developed as an evaluative measure. Other tools, such as the PEDI,[22,23] have been tested for their responsiveness to change and as such can be classified as evaluative tests.

Can one tool be used to discriminate, predict, and evaluate change?

It is possible for a tool to have discriminatory, predictive, and evaluative capabilities, but such a tool is more an exception than a rule. Discriminatory tools are usually developed from a cross-sectional sample, which means that the participants are only tested once. For the test to meet the criteria for an evaluative measure, the children must be tested at least twice over a period of time (longitudinal). This is an important distinction. A few studies have examined the evaluative validity (responsiveness) of discriminatory tools after they have been published. Examples are the first edition of the PDMS and Bayley,[24] the PDMS-2, and the PEDI.[22] Many more discriminatory measures have not been tested. Some test developers have combined cross-sectional with longitudinal designs and were therefore able to evaluate the tool's capacity to discriminate, predict outcome, and evaluate change. One such tool is the TIMP.[15,25,26]

What does the law require regarding nondiscriminatory evaluations and assessments?

Evaluation and assessment procedures must be nondiscriminatory. Sec. 303.320(a)(3) says:

> *All evaluations and assessments of the child and family must be conducted by qualified personnel, in a nondiscriminatory manner, in the child's or family's native language (as appropriate), and selected and administered so as not to be racially or culturally discriminatory.*

This provision suggests that therapists must understand the limitations of the tests they use to determine eligibility in terms of cultural competency and language proficiency, and seek additional resources when needed. Because the instructions for tests such as the BSID-III or BDI-2 are in English, the use of interpreters can make a difference in the child's overall performance, score on the test, and ultimately in eligibility. By understanding the instructions and the purpose of testing, caregivers can also help motivate the child during testing. A chapter by Garcia-Coll and Magnusson[27] presents a comprehensive overview of the relationship between cultural differences and child outcome.

Many of the tools used to assess children have not demonstrated cultural validity, suggesting the need for physical therapists to exercise a great deal of caution when interpreting the results of the tests with culturally diverse populations. They also should consider information gathered through interviews with caregivers, such as a child's developmental history, and medical history, if available. According to Hui and Triandis,[28] the process of cultural validity entails determination of whether a measure accurately reflects a given construct even when used with different social groups. These authors assert that for a measure to be considered culturally valid, a construct (eg, self-help) should have the same meaning to other populations: (1) at a conceptual level, (2) in how it is operationally defined, (3) in the items used to test that construct, and (4) in the meaning of the scaled score. Therefore evaluation of the cultural validity of a measure requires 4 levels of analyses, which can be accomplished through additional research. Cultural validity is more than the inclusion of children from diverse populations in the normative sample.

How is "evaluation" defined in Part B?

Part B does not distinguish between evaluation and assessment. Sec. 300.15 states:

> *Evaluation means procedures used in accordance with Sec. 300.304-300.311 to determine whether a child has a disability and the nature and extent of the special education and related services that the child needs.*

This definition of evaluation describes 2 distinct purposes and processes. The first purpose and process is to determine if a student has a disability, which is similar to the Part C definition of evaluation. If, through this first process, a student is found to have a disability (see Chapter 3 for categories of disability), the second purpose is to "determine the nature and extent of special education and related services that the child needs."

What is the responsibility of a physical therapist in the evaluation to determine if a child has a disability?

Physical therapists can contribute in 2 ways to evaluations that determine if a student has a disability, as defined under Part B. In states that have decided to use the "developmental delay" category for students ages 3 through 9 or some subset of this age span (an option under federal regulations), physical therapists can assist in identifying and documenting a student's delays, usually in motor areas. This process is similar to determining children's eligibility for Part C programs. Physical therapists' evaluations also may contribute to identifying and documenting disability categories for students older than the appropriate age for the "developmental delay" category. In some states, for example, determination of a child's eligibility under the "orthopedic impairment" category requires an evaluation of motor functioning by a physical therapist or occupational therapist. Other states have other requirements that could involve physical therapy evaluations, both to determine a child's disability and the child's need for special education and related services because of the disability.

Are physical therapists required to use specific tests or types of tests to determine a student's eligibility for special education and related services?

Part B allows the use of a variety of tests or approaches to determine if the student is eligible for special services and related services:

> *Sec. 300.304 Evaluation procedures.*
>
> *(b) (1) Use a variety of assessment tools and strategies to gather relevant functional, developmental, and academic information about the child, including information provided by the parent, that may assist in determining-*
>
> *(i) Whether the child is a child with a disability under Sec 300.8; and*
>
> *(ii) The content of the child's IEP, including information related to enabling the child to be involved in and progress in the general education curriculum (or for a preschool child, to participate in appropriate activities);*
>
> *(2) Not use a single measure or assessment as the sole criterion for determining whether a child is a child with a disability and for determining an appropriate educational program for the child; and*
>
> *(3) Use technically sound instruments that may assess the relative contribution of cognitive and behavioral factors, in addition to physical or developmental factors.*
>
> *(c) (1) (i) Are selected and administered so as to not be discriminatory on a racial or cultural basis;*
>
> *(ii) Are provided and administered in the child's native language or other mode of communication and in the form most likely to yield accurate information on what the child knows and can do academically, developmentally, and functionally, unless it is clearly not feasible to so provide or administer;*
>
> *(iii) Are used for the purposes for which the assessment or measure are valid and reliable;*
>
> *(iv) Are administered by trained and knowledgeable personnel; and*
>
> *(v) Are administered in accordance with any instructions provided by the producer of the assessments.*

Similarly, Sec. 300.304(c)(3) states:

> *Assessments are selected and administered so as best to ensure that if an assessment is administered to a child with impaired sensory, manual, or speaking skills, the assessment results accurately reflect the child's aptitude or achievement level or whatever other factors the test purports to measure, rather than reflecting the child's impaired sensory, manual, or speaking skills (unless those skills are the factors the test purports to measure).*

IDEA also requires that:

Sec. 300.304(c)(1) Evaluation and assessment materials used to assess a child under this part—

(iv) Are administered by trained and knowledgeable personnel

(v) Are administered in accordance with any instructions provided by the producer of the assessments.

(vi) Are used for the purposes for which the assessment or measure are valid and reliable; …

These regulations mean that physical therapists should not only understand the psychometric properties of the tests that are useful for helping to determine eligibility or program planning, but also know how to evaluate them. The provision that the assessment accurately reflects that child's aptitude or achievement level underscores the importance of reading test manuals and following the directions specified for administration of test items. Modifications of standardized procedures, if needed, should be reported and taken into considerations when interpreting test scores. An example is a child who needs 4-5 trials to pass items on the PDMS II when the manual specifies the maximum of 3 trials. Indeed the need for high repetitions may indicate that the child has deficits in domains other than motor.

Based on these regulations physical therapists, to the best of their abilities, must not only ensure that students understand test instructions, but also that testing procedures are not culturally or racially biased. The regulations also suggest that in addition to assessments being conducted in a language that the child understands, the tests selected should not be culturally or racially biased. Cultural validity is described in the previous section.

Many of the published tests that physical therapists use were developed for specific purposes and for children within a specific age range. Tests that were designed to identify children with motor delays, for example, may not be valid measures of change following intervention or use with children with severe disabilities. Another common misuse of tests is to administer instruments designed for infants and young children, such as the BSID-II, to older children with severe motor impairments. Information obtained from misused tests serves no valid purpose.

Do physical therapists have to document students' age-equivalent scores?

IDEA does not require documentation of a student's "motor age" or age-equivalent scores in any other areas of development, except perhaps for eligibility purposes for children in the developmental delay category. As discussed in Chapter 6, when writing an individualized education program, it is much more useful to describe what a student can and cannot do in personally meaningful terms than to report age-equivalent scores. This is especially true when students' age-equivalent scores are far below their chronological ages. Knowing that a 6-year-old student has a gross motor age-equivalent score of 5 months and a fine motor age-equivalent score of 8 months, for example, tells us nothing that helps to plan an appropriate program for the child.

Are failed items on developmental tests good for IFSP or IEP goals?

It depends. As discussed in chapters 5 and 6, which describe individualized family service plans and individualized education programs, respectively, programs must be developed to accomplish individually meaningful outcomes or goals. For infants and toddlers with developmental delays, items such as attaining independent sitting, crawling, and walking without hands held may appropriate and tend to also be among the family's expected goals. Failed items on measures that assess the child's skills in specific settings, such as PEDI or SFA may also be appropriately targeted for intervention. On the other hand, failed items on norm- or criterion-referenced developmental tests are rarely appropriate for children with moderate to severe disabilities who are unlikely to progress far enough along a developmental sequence to accomplish skills useful to older children or adults.

What other methods can physical therapists use?

The assessment methods discussed thus far have focused on quantitative measures (tests). Part C and Part B require using a variety of procedures, including informed opinion based on the use of qualitative measures (interviews and observation). Physical therapists tend to use interviews during the initial stages of the assessment process. When done well, interviews can allow the physical therapist to gain insight into children's worlds or to understand their perspectives in ways that a questionnaire or test cannot. Examples are recurrent themes presented in the information that parents share during the interview, themes that highlight the importance of family values such as communication, education and knowledge, participation in community activities, and strategies that the child and family have used. Interviews also allow great flexibility in how and what information is gathered (structured, semi-structured, or unstructured). To a good listener, information gathered through interviews can be valuable in guiding the assessment process and even selecting appropriate tools for further investigation.

Observation is another qualitative method that is widely used to gather information during assessments. Like an interview, observation can allow one to gain insight about a setting or interactions among individuals, and can allow one to formulate ideas about how the phenomena observed interact (context).

The qualitative approach to assessment or information gathering is not without challenges, particularly when it comes to interpreting results. Interviews also require skill.[8] In their chapter on interpreting interviews, Fontana and Frey[29] point out that many people think they can do interviews, talking to people from all walks of life with ease, but often forget about that the type of information obtained lies in the art of interviewing. Corcoran[10] raises 2 fundamental questions that are related to the use of qualitative methods in measurement or assessment — the question of knowing whether "the right questions are being asked" and how we "ensure that we have conducted and interpreted our observations and interviews accurately."[10(p57)] A detailed discussion of interview methods is beyond the scope of this chapter. There are many texts on interviewing, such as chapters by Corcoran[10] and Fontana and Frey.[29] These authors caution against interviewers' perceptions that they are neutral or unbiased when it comes to interpretation, and that when faced with a mountain of notes, the interviewer chooses what to report or not report (interpretive validity). The interviewer role is particularly consequential when used for assessments with diverse populations.

Physical therapists who use interviews must make sure that important components of the interview process are taken into consideration, for example the types of questions that would generate the most pertinent information, agreement on how to interpret the information once it is gathered, the process of developing working hypotheses, and criteria for selection of follow-up test and measures. Although generating working hypotheses is an important step, these hypotheses can pose the greatest challenges to interpreting information gathered through interviews. Every working hypothesis must be tested and confirmed or refuted through additional testing. Examples of working hypotheses that are based on an interview with a parent of Jay, a 4-year-old child with autism who is in a preschool program, may be: (1) The amount of information the family has received about their child's condition underlies the parents' difficulty in coping, or (2) uncertainty in predicting, and increasing difficulty in managing Jay's behavior outside the home, is central to his mother's sense of diminishing capacity to carry out her roles as a mother, wife, daughter, and sibling.

When relying on the observation method, therapists need to remember that factors such as observer and setting bias, observer effects, and whether or not a person is aware that they are being observed can all affect the reliability of observations and validity of the conclusions drawn. Portney and Watkins[30] and Patton[31] propose several methods, such as participant observer or observer participants. All attempt to capture the real experience of the individual (in this case the child in various setting and family), but this can be difficult to implement in some settings. Physical therapists need to be mindful that these challenges alter the reality they are trying to capture and should exercise caution in how they interpret the information gathered through observation.

What are the advantages and disadvantages of using quantitative or qualitative methods of assessment?

Qualitative methods capture context and focus on processes and meanings—the socially constructed nature of reality and the meaning assigned to experiences. In contrast, the quantitative approach focuses on products such as quantity, amount, intensity, or frequency. Both capture reality or a person's point of view. Using qualitative measures may help the physical therapist get closer to the problem through detailed interviews and observations. On the other hand, interpretations that are based on qualitative methods can be unreliable, value-laden, and highly subjective. Both approaches can be flawed. It is hard to capture reality, particularly that of another person, or the meaning of another's action, or intention. It is also difficult to give objective accounts of the phenomenon under observation, even if the observations are made in their natural environments. Regardless of approach, we need to keep in mind that our previous understandings and prejudices shape the interpretive process (this is often referred to in qualitative research as hermeneutics).[30] Qualitative methods do not have measures, such as the standard error of measurement, that can be used when interpreting tests results to accommodate observer/testee biases or errors.

Combining qualitative and quantitative approaches appears more advantageous than using either method alone. Using Jay's example and the working hypotheses described previously, the 2 approaches can be combined in the following manner: If difficulty in anticipating or predicting Jay's behavior appears to also be at the heart of what is hypothesized to be a "threat" to the family's engagement in social activities, theoretical models such as the Social Communication, Emotional Regulation, and Transactional Support (SCERTS)[32] could be used to guide the selection of assessment tools (eg, the Sensory Profile). Regardless of the method or approach used, physical therapists should be mindful of the importance of consistency in how information is gathered during assessment. Consistency extends beyond reliability of tools to the question of efficacy, and helps address questions about the credibility of interpretations, Although IDEA offers flexibility in methods used to assess children, judicious use of the methods and tools is the physical therapist's responsibility.

What is a good way to approach assessment and program planning?

Theoretical models and frameworks are valuable in guiding systematic assessments and evaluations. Two different physical therapists who assess the same child may come up with different findings, and those differences could be a function of the theoretical model and framework they use. The social science literature tends to use models to describe a representation of ideas in a specific relationship. Frameworks, on the other hand, tend to be used to describe a structure that comprises various elements. A framework can consist of several models.

Models and frameworks provide a common and standard way of describing information gathered from observations, tests, or interviews and provide a standard way of thinking about where to begin, define what exactly one should asses, decide what to do with the information gathered, and help us interpret assessment findings. Similarly, a model used by physical therapists should guide how they structure an assessment for children with disabilities by helping answer questions that are related to: How to begin and why; what kinds of questions to ask, and in what order; who should be informants; what criteria should be used to select informants; how much weight should be placed on the various informants; what tools to use to gather information and why; and how should the assessment findings be interpreted. Models and frameworks do not inform how to treat children, nor do they guarantee success of assessment or intervention.

The literature presents a variety of models such as Gentile's model of skill acquisition,[33] Bronfenbrenner's[34] ecological model of human development, or the transactional model of development by Sameroff and Chandler (1975) and described by Sameroff and Fiese,[35] the SCERTS model developed by Prizant and colleagues,[32] and the participation model of leisure and recreation developed by King and colleagues.[36] Physical therapy has used the disablement model developed initially by Nagi[37] to guide assessment and intervention described in the APTA *Guide to Physical Therapist Practice*.[38]

More recently, the framework that has increasingly gained attention is the *International Classification of Functioning, Disability and Health: ICF*[39] developed by the World Health Organization (WHO). The development of the ICF stemmed from the need to find a common language for practitioners to use internationally to describe health and disability. In *Towards a Common Language for Functioning, Disability and Health*,[40] WHO states that the ICF "is a scientific tool for consistent, internationally comparable information about the experience of health and disability."[(p5)] The ICF is considered a biopsychosocial model because it combines major conceptual models of disability: the medical and social models. The focus in the ICF is on the components of health versus the consequences of disease, as has been the case with previous models developed by WHO.[40]

What are the components of the ICF framework?

The ICF consists of 3 levels of functioning: body structures and functions, activity, and participation; and 2 factors: personal and environmental factors (Figure 4-1). Taken together, these components are consistent with the IDEA 2004 requirement for comprehensive assessments and evaluation of personal and environmental factors that may facilitate or hinder the children's ability to perform and participate in expected or desired activities. The structure of the ICF offers qualifiers for each level of functioning, such as extent and nature of change in body functions and structure, and performance and capability in activities and participation. The environmental factors component gives consideration to attitudes, support, and technology. Although the ICF expresses each component in positive terms, it also uses negative language to describe barriers or constraints that contribute to disability. For example, terms such as *impairments in body functions and structures* and *limitations in activities and participation* are used to describe and identify personal and environmental factors that serve as barriers at any of the 3 levels.

Figure 4-1. Interactions between the levels and factors of the International Classification of Functioning, Disability, and Health (ICF) model.[39]

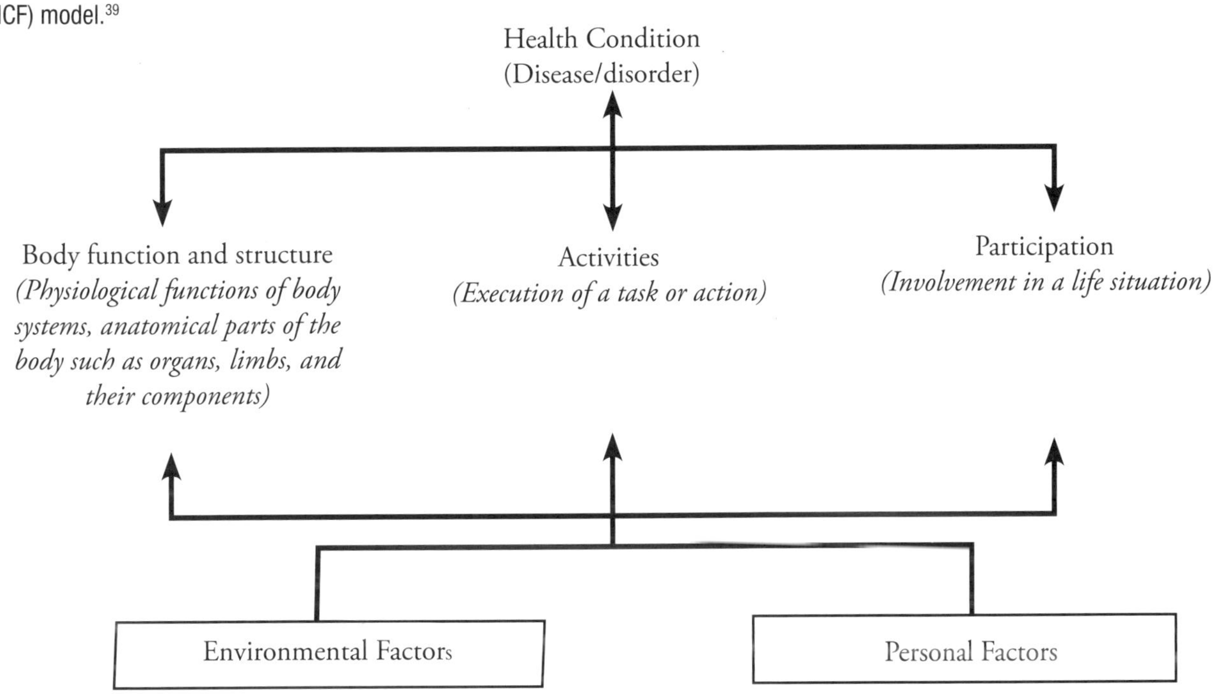

Any of the 3 levels of functioning can be used as a port of entry for assessment; however, beginning at the participation level seems most logical. First, most of the presenting problems that parents and teachers use as reasons to consult with or refer the child for physical therapy tend to be at the participation level, such as access related to constraints in mobility. Second, participation in activities such as caregiving or recreation is the ultimate goal for health and function for most children and their families. Third, participation is contextual and provides a broader picture of an individual's capacity and capability, such as the ability to complete daily tasks. One principle of the ICF model is that an individual's ability to participate is inextricably linked with environmental factors. Because relationships among participation, activity, and body functions and structures tend to be linear, evaluation and assessment that proceeds from participation to the activity level to body functions and structures are likely to link the levels in a meaningful way. For example, some limitations at the participation level may be due to environmental factors and some may be directly linked to limitations at the activity level.

Constraints in body functions and structures may underlie limitations at the activity level, making this the last step in assessment. A family may be concerned about the safety of a 20-month-old child who falls frequently (limited participation). Evaluation of walking in and around the home and the results of the locomotion and object manipulation sections the PDMS II may reveal that he can only walk safely on level surfaces, but cannot walk fast, backwards, and up or down the stairs, or kick a ball (activity limitations). Assessment of body structures and functions may reveal visual-motor deficits as major constraints underlying the activity and participation limitations. The sequence described focuses the scope of assessment to the presenting problem or desired goals, and reduces redundancy.

Constraints in body functions and structures, however, do not always lead to limitations at the activity level, and limitations at the activity level inconsistently contribute to limitations at the participation level. Similarly, interventions targeted at one level inconsistently affect other levels. Physical therapy traditionally has focused on assessing impairments in body functions and structures, such as muscle weakness or paralysis, poor control of posture and balance, joint range limitations, abnormal muscle contraction, fatigue, and other problems that result from abnormalities in body functions; however, not all of these may constrain the child's activity and participation. Little evidence exists that intervention targeted solely at this level is effective for improving function of children with developmental disabilities. Sometimes changing environmental factors, such as though the use of assistive technology, can improve performance without changing impairments in body structures. Several texts give examples of how to apply the ICF to children.[8,39,41] A case example plan of how physical therapists can use the ICF to assess and evaluate older children is presented at the end of this chapter.

What types of assessments are useful to plan programs aimed at improving participation?

Program planning is a process whereby assessment findings (eg, participation, activity limitations, and body functions and structures) are used to guide goals and intervention plans. Tools such as the School Function Assessment (SFA) and the Pediartric Evaluation of Disability Inventory (PEDI) can be used to obtain information about a child's abilities from a parent, teacher, or other informant who knows the child well. Another useful tool is the Canadian Occupational Performance Measure (COPM),[42] which was designed for occupational therapists, but also can help physical therapists to identify and measure individually meaningful goals for children. The COPM focuses on children's occupations and asks children to identify important problem areas and rate their ability to perform tasks in the areas. Young children between the ages of 5 and 9 may be able to play a role in identifying goals, depending on the child's cognitive level. Another tool that can be used with this group is the Perceived Efficacy and Goal Setting System (PEGS), a system that allows children 5-8 years old to identify and prioritize their own goals.[43] Missiuna and Pollock[44] found that although parents and children identified similar goals, the priority of the goals were different. The PEGS is still in the process of being further validated.

How can physical therapists evaluate the outcomes of their interventions in early intervention and school programs?

Both Parts C and B require periodic review of children's IFSP or IEP to determine progress and to inform action plan based on the outcome. Part C requires monitoring of the IFSP at least every 6 months.

Sec. 303.342 Procedures for IFSP development, review, and evaluation.

(b) Periodic review.

(1) A review of the IFSP for a child and the child's family must be conducted every six months, or more frequently if conditions warrant, or if the family requests such a review. The purpose of the periodic review is to determine—

(i) The degree to which progress toward achieving the outcomes is being made; and

(ii) Whether modifications or revision of the outcomes or services is necessary.

(c) Annual meeting to evaluate the IFSP. A meeting must be conducted to evaluate the IFSP for a child and the child's family, and, as appropriate, to revise its provisions. The results of any current evaluations conducted under Sec. 303.320, and other information available from the assessment of the service needs must be used in determining what services are needed and will be provided.

Part B requires at least an annual review:

Sec. 300.324 Development, review, and revisions of IEP:

(6)(b) Review and revision of IEPs. Each public agency must ensure that the IEP team:

(i) Reviews the child's IEP periodically, but not less than annually, to determine whether the annual goals for the child are being achieved; and

(ii) Revises the IEP, as appropriate to address:

(A) Any lack of expected progress toward the annual goals described in Sec. 300.320(a)(2), and in the general curriculum, if appropriate;

(B) The results of reevaluations conducted under Sec. 300.303;

(C) Information about the child provided to, or by, the parents, as described in Sec. 300.305(a)(2);

(D) The child's anticipated needs; or

(E) Other matters

To assess progress or the outcome of intervention one needs an evaluative measure. In early intervention and educational settings physical therapists use goals on the IFSP and IEP extensively to assess the outcomes of their interventions. Universal to the literature and research on measuring change is the assumption that interventions are based on assessment findings, which are also linked to goals (or outcomes).The advantages are that goals are individualized, based on the child's potential abilities, easy to assess in educational and other natural environments, and may be developed to focus on all the levels of the ICF. For these reasons goals are useful and allow therapists to use multiple sources of data in making decisions pertaining to intervention and outcomes for each individual child. When appropriately written in observable and measurable formats, goals can meet the reliability and validity requirements for evaluative measures outlined by Guyatt et al [21] and Kirshner et al.[11]

Goals as evaluative measures, however, are also limited and present a challenge when used to evaluate the effectiveness of interventions at an individual level, but more so for groups of children at a program level or across programs. The difficulty in accurately predicting the exact level of attainment of goals within a given period by each child and the difficulty in scaling criteria are some factors that may threaten the credibility of using goals to determine the effectiveness of interventions. Accurate predictions allow one to determine whether or not a child with a specific disability can meet the goals within a given period. *Scaling* refers to breaking down goals into measurable units, such as the "complete," "partially complete," "cannot do" criteria for the PEDI, or the 5 levels in Goal Attainment Scaling (GAS).[45] Scaling informs one about the degree of ability or completeness of performance. What is often overlooked when using scaling criteria such as 3 out of 4 trials is what is being scaled and what each level represents.

Criteria such as 3/5 times, or 3/5 trials suggest that 3/5 is better than 2/5 and better than 1/5. For this to be true, each trial or number should represent a threshold for minimal significant change or a different level of performance, as in GAS. Another measurement dilemma is interpreting outcomes that use of the number of goals achieved as an outcome measure, for example, meeting 4 out of 7 goals. Physical therapists should practice scaling their goals in such a way that changes in the criteria represent a clinically (or functionally) significant change, and may find resources by Palisano et al,[45] Forbes,[46] and Cusick et al[47] to be helpful.

Bias associated with the method used to judge attainment of the goals is another drawback. To minimize bias when comparing groups of children enrolled in a program, a physical therapist other than the treating physical therapist could rate the goals. This is particularly important when goals are used during program evaluation as indicators of quality assurance, productivity, or overall program effectiveness. Having another physical therapist rate the goals may not always be practical. Procedures for observations of the goals should be decided during IEP or IFSP meetings.

Using age-equivalent scores (AE) to determine the outcome of intervention presents problems similar to interpretation of IFSP and IEP goals. For example, a 3-month AE score gain over a period of 6 months may be good for a 24-month-old child whose pretest age equivalent score was 3 months, but not for another 24-month-old child whose pretest age equivalent score was 15 months. Also a change of 2 or 3 months AE over a 12-month period is difficult to interpret even for an individual child.

Criterion testing may be an excellent way of measuring progress over time in a standard environment. Natural environments tend to have a great deal of variability and therefore make it harder to evaluate progress over time. For this purpose, tools such as the PEDI and GMFM might be an appropriate assessment tool to measure changes in participation and activities over time. Ketellar[23] found that of 17 described measures only 2, the GMFM and the PEDI, meet the criteria for reliability and validity with respect to responsiveness to change.

A tool that is rarely used systematically in evaluating outcomes of intervention is parent questionnaires, despite results that demonstrated that parents can be objective in their judgments. Russell and associates[48] used parent and physical therapist ratings as an external criterion measure in their development of the GMFM. Parents made concurrent judgments about motor function independent of physical therapists treating the children on whom the GMFM was administered. PTs who plan to use parent ratings should keep in mind that the observation tool must at least demonstrate the same psychometric properties as other measures in terms of reliability and validity.

SUMMARY

The process of assessment and evaluation as outlined in Parts C and B of IDEA requires systematic information gathering. The choice of assessment tools and interpretation of the findings is left up to qualified professionals like physical therapists. Understanding the psychometric properties of tests used and how to interpret information gathered using quantitative or qualitative methods is paramount in ensuring that children who are eligible for Part C or Part B services are not overlooked. Frameworks such as the ICF are helpful in organizing the assessment process, ensuring that assessments are comprehensive, and in maintaining consistency in how information is gathered. Physical therapists should not only be familiar with the criteria for eligibility and service provision in their states, but must also ensure that the criteria and tools used are not biased against children and families from diverse backgrounds, including those with disabilities.

Case Example of Assessment and Evaluation Plan Using the ICF

Rene is a 6-year-old girl with spastic quadriplegia. According to the mother, she was born at term age following an uncomplicated pregnancy. Her neonatal period was unremarkable. At the age of 4 months Rene developed seizures that could not be successfully controlled with medication until she was 1 year of age. The CT scan results at age 2 revealed brain atrophy, a porencephalic cyst on the left side, and slightly enlarged ventricles. At that time Rene was enrolled in an early intervention program where she had received weekly physical therapy, occupational therapy, speech therapy, and services from a child development specialist. At age 5 years a derotation osteotomy of her right femur and bilateral adductor muscles release were performed due to severe adductor muscles spasticity and hamstring muscle shortening. Following the removal of a hip spica cast she was fitted with ankle-foot orthoses, and a power wheelchair was ordered for her. Rene is now 5 years, 8 months old. She will be starting school in the fall and is scheduled to receive a comprehensive evaluation and assessment by a team of professionals from the school. Rene's mother is anxious about this transition and wants Rene to "do well."

Assessment at the Participation Level

Ability to perform and participate in the new environment (school) seems to be central to this referral; therefore, the assessment process would begin at the participation level. Because transition is a concern, information gathered at this level would include Rene's and her family's expectations for successful transition to a new school, her previous intervention team's perception of her level of functioning (baseline data), and how Rene's participation has changed over time. Tools used: interview and tools such as Perceived Efficacy and Goal Setting System (PEGS)[43] or the Canadian Occupational Performance Measure (COPM).[44] PEGS is a system that allows children 5-8 years of age to identify and prioritize their own goals. The COPM focuses on children's occupations, and asks children to identify important problem areas and to rate their ability to perform tasks in the areas. Other areas of participation may include ability to complete classroom activities (with focus on autonomy, enjoyment, and sense of fulfillment, in addition to performance), use of language and ability to express wants and needs, interpersonal interactions and relationships, and available environmental supports. To assess communication and interpersonal interactions and relationships, observational measures such as event sampling (how often during timed observations) or interval recording (how long during timed observations) can also be useful for baseline data.

One may also choose to observe Rene in her classroom, paying attention to the effect of the environment on her alertness and interactions, noting any supports that she requires to be successful, and the social context of Rene's classroom participation by noting the teachers' and others students' attitudes toward her. As Rosenbaum and Stewart[40] stated, "the social and cultural environment must be considered in assessment and intervention, because we know that the attitudes, values, and beliefs of others affect a child's participation in daily activities."[(p9)]

Access is key to Rene's participation in the new setting (school). Therefore assessment of participation would also include mobility: accessing the school building (bathroom, cafeteria, and playground), traveling between classrooms, and independence and autonomy in getting on/off the bus. Methods of data collection could include observation and use of setting specific tools as the School Function Assessment.[49] The ICF qualifier scale of performance and capacity as outlined on the ICF checklist found on the Web site http://www3.who.int/icf/icftemplate.cfm would also be appropriate, but may need to be modified. Use of the SFA, a judgment-based assessment tool, is valuable in facilitating a collaborative approach to planning a program of appropriate supports for Rene; however, this would be appropriate if scheduled after school has started. To increase the accuracy of the scores, the developers of the SFA recommend using respondents who are familiar with the student, who have observed the student engaged in the activities being assessed by the tool, and who understand the type of supports that are usually provided to the student's same age/grade peers and how those students would typically perform those same tasks.[50] Note the blending of the personal and environmental factors of the participation level of the ICF and the use of qualitative and quantitative methods in this example.

Assessment and evaluation at the activity and body function and structure levels would not be initiated until concerns or limitations in Rene's participation have been identified and working hypotheses have been formulated. This is particularly important because some of the barriers to Rene's participation may be related to environmental factors. The results of the SFA, on the other hand, would provide information about Rene's independence in performing functional tasks that support participation in school. The results of the PEDI or SFA could also be used to determine activity barriers to participation. The PEDI results would provide information about Rene's level of independence in self help, mobility, and social function at home. Progressing in this order may represent a shift from how many physical therapists have approached assessment and evaluation.

Mobility. Depending on the results of the PEDI or SFA and working hypotheses, assessment of mobility related barriers to participation would ensue. Assessment of mobility at the activity level would occur with Rene using her power wheelchair in the classroom, the playground, bathroom, cafeteria, and during transitions. These are activities all students actively participate in during a school day. One could record how she performed in each setting by using a simple rating scale (0 = needs assistance, 1 = completes with supervision, 2 = independent), or use the number of errors (eg, running into walls, furniture, etc) in a given distance (eg, in the hallway), or speed (timing). Information gained from such observations could be used as a baseline to monitor changes in Rene's ability to control her power wheelchair.

Transfers. Ability to transfer may also be hypothesized as a barrier to participation. Assessment at this level would focus on observation of how Rene performs transfers in the bathroom, classroom, or gym. Task analysis and videography can help the physical therapist and the team identify which environments or environmental supports produce the preferred combination of successes (eg, Rene is able to maintain more standing for transfers when using a grab bar to pull up, rather than push up from the wheelchair). Note that these data would be valuable for establishing goals related to the self-care activity of toileting as well.

The evaluation team could also collaborate on the task and tool portions of the Student-centered, Environmentally useful, and Tasks-focused Tool (SETT) system[51] to determine classroom expectations and activities that Rene will have. Activities could include the following: (1) level of independence using power wheelchair when accessing transportation (if using bus), navigating within the school environment, and access to outdoor play equipment; (2) Rene's ability to use alternative means of mobility within classroom when not in power chair (including transfers and floor mobility or walking as appropriate); and (3) the need for augmentative communication.

Assessment at the Body Function and Structure Level

Again, evaluation at the body function and structure would not be initiated until concerns or limitations are noted in Rene's performance (activity level). Movement analysis is valuable for the assessment of body functions and structures that are believed or hypothesized to contribute to the limitations observed during assessment at the activity and participation levels. Therefore, movement analysis should enable one to determine the nature of limitations at these levels. Information gained from the movement analysis may uncover the reasons for those mobility constraints. If Rene exhibited excessive hip and knee flexion during transfers, for example, an assessment of hip range of motion (ROM), muscle strength, and spasticity might be appropriate. The following tools could be useful: goniometer for ROM, manual muscle testing or hand-held dynamometer for muscle strength, and the modified Ashworth scale for muscle spasticity. If one hypothesized that pain was an underlying constraint, a pain scale could be used. These measures could provide valuable information on the nature and extent of impairments in body functions and structures that limit Rene's specific activities and desired or expected areas of participation. Note that these assessments may be undertaken only if they are believed to be the underlying constraints.

SUMMARY

In summary, this example of an assessment plan is guided by the ICF framework, combines qualitative and quantitative approaches and measures, and relies on the expertise of the therapists (qualified personnel). The concern that Rene's family initially expressed is used to inform the assessment plan. The top-down approach emphasizes identifying participation and activity performance first and then the underlying factors that may interfere with them.

REFERENCES

1. Folio RM, Fewell R. *Peabody Developmental Motor Scales.* 2nd ed. Austin, TX: Pro-Ed; 2000.
2. Dwyer CA. Cut scores and testing: statistics, judgment, truth, and error. *Psychol Assess.* 1996;8:360-362.
3. Andersson LL. Appropriate and inappropriate interpretation and use of test scores in early intervention. *J Early Intervent.* 2004;27:55-68.
4. Fletcher RH, Fletcher SW, Wagner EH. *Clinical Epidemiology: The Essentials.* 3rd ed. Baltimore, MD: Williams & Wilkins; 1996.
5. Aylward GP. Conceptual issues in developmental screening and assessment. *J Dev Behav Pediatric.* 1997;18:340-349.
6. Russell DJ, Rosenbaum PL, Avery LM, Lane M. *Gross Motor Function Measure (GMFM-66 & GMFM-88) User's Manual.* London, England: Mac Keith Press; 2002.
7. Haley SM, Coster WJ, Ludlow LH, Haltiwanger J, Andrellos P. *Pediatric Valuation of Disability Inventory (PEDI): Development, Standardization, and Administration Manual.* Boston, MA: PEDI Research Group; 1992.
8. Palisano RJ, Campbell SK, Harris SR. Evidence-based decision making in pediatric physical therapy. In: Campbell S, Vander Linden D, Palisano R, eds. *Physical Therapy for Children.* St Louis, MO: Saunders Elsevier; 2006:3-32.
9. Mattingly C, Fleming M. *Clinical Reasoning: Forms of Inquiry in a Therapeutic Practice.* Philadelphia, PA: FA Davis; 1994.
10. Corcoran M. Using qualitative measurement methods to understand occupational performance. In: Law M, Baum C, Dunn W, eds. *Measuring Occupational Performance: Supporting Best Practice in Occupational Therapy.* Thorofare, NJ: Slack; 2001:57-64.
11. Kirshner B, Guyatt GH. A methodologic framework for assessing health indices. *J Chronic Dis.* 1985;38:27-36.
12. Bayley N. *Bayley Scales of Infant and Toddler Development.* 3rd ed. San Antonio, TX: Psychological Corporation; 2005.
13. Piper MC, Darrah J. *Motor Assessment of the Developing Infant.* Philadelphia, Pa: WB Saunders; 1993.
14. Newborg J. *Battelle Developmental Inventory.* 2nd ed. Itasca, IL: Riverside Publishing; 2005.
15. Campbell SK, Kolobe THA, Wright BD, Linacre JM. Validity of the Test of Infant Motor Performance for prediction of 6-, 9-, and 12-month scores on the Alberta Infant Motor Scale. *Dev Med Child Neurol.* 2002;44:263-272.
16. Parks S. *Hawaii Early Learning Profile.* Palo Alto, CA: Vort Corporation; 1992.
17. Darrah J, Piper M, Watt M-J. Assessment of gross motor skills of at-risk infants: predictive validity of the Alberta Infant Motor Scale. *Dev Med Child Neurol.* 1998a;40:485-491.
18. Harris SR, Daniels, LE. Content validity of the Harris Infant Neuromotor Test. *Phys Ther.* 1996;76:727-737.
19. Campbell SK, Swanlund A, Smith E, Liao P-J, Zawacki L. Validity of the TIMPSI for estimating concurrent performance on the Test of Infant Motor Performance. *Pediatr Phys Ther.* 2008;20(1):3-10.
20. Bricker D, Squires J; with assistance from Mounts L, Potter L, Nickel R, Twombly E, Farrell J. *Ages & Stages Questionnaires® (ASQ): A Parent-Completed, Child-Monitoring System.* Baltimore, MD: Paul H. Brookes Publishing Company; 1999.
21. Guyatt G, Walter S, Norman G. Measuring change over time: assessing the usefulness of evaluative instruments. *J Chronic Dis.* 1987;40:171-178.
22. Iyer LV, Haley SM, Watkins MP, Dumas HM. Establishing minimal clinically important differences for scores on the Pediatric Evaluation of Disability: inventory for inpatient rehabilitation. *Phys Ther.* 2003;83:888-898.
23. Ketelaar M, Vermeer A, Helders P. Functional motor abilities of children with cerebral palsy: a systematic literature review of assessment measures. *Clin Rehabil.* 1998;5:369–380.
24. Kolobe THA, Palisano R, Stratford P. Comparison of two outcome measures for infants with cerebral palsy and infants with motor delays. *Phys Ther.* 1998;78:1062-1072.
25. Campbell SK, Hedeker D. Validity of the Test of Infant Motor Performance for discriminating among infants with varying risk for poor motor outcome. *J Pediatr.* 2001;139:546-551.
26. Kolobe TH, Bulanda M, Susman L. Predicting motor outcome at preschool age for infants tested at 7, 30, and 90 days after term age using the Test of Infant Motor Performance. *Phys Ther.* 2004;84:1144-1156.
27. Garcia-Coll C, Magnusson K. Cultural differences as sources of developmental vulnerabilities and resources. In: Shonkoff J, Meisels S, eds. *Handbook of Early Childhood Intervention.* 2nd ed. Cambridge: Cambridge University Press; 2000:94-114.
28. Hui CH, Triandis HC. Measurement in cross-cultural psychology: a review and comparison strategies. *J Cross-cultural Psychol.* 1985;16:131-152.
29. Fontana, A, Frey JH. Interviewing: the art of science. In: Denzin NK, Lincoln YS, eds. *Collecting and Interpreting Qualitative Materials.* Thousand Oaks, CA: SAGE Publications; 1998:47-77.
30. Portney LG, Watkins MP. *Foundations of Clinical Research: Applications to Practice.* 2nd ed. Upper Saddle River, NJ: Prentice Hall Health; 2000.
31. Patton MQ. *Qualitative Evaluation and Research Methods.* 2nd ed. Newbury Park, CA: Sage; 1990:277-368.
32. Prizant B, Wetherby A, Rubin E, Laurent A. The SCERTS Model: a transactional, family-centered approach to enhancing communication and socio-emotional abilities of children with Autism Spectrum Disorder. *Inf Young Child.* 2003;16:296-316.

33. Gentile AM. Skill acquisition: action, movement, and neuromotor processes. In: Carr JC, Shepherd R, eds. *Movement Science: Foundations for Physical Therapy in Rehabilitation.* 2nd ed. Gaithersburg, MD: Aspen; 2000:111-187.

34. Bronfenbrenner U. Ecology of the family as a context for human development research perspectives. *Dev Psychol.* 1986;22:723-742.

35. Sameroff AJ, Fiese BH. Transactional regulation: the development ecology of early intervention. In: Shonkoff J, Meisels S, eds. *Handbook of Early Childhood Intervention.* 2nd ed. New York, NY: Cambridge University Press; 2000:135-159.

36. King G, King S, Rosenbaum P, et al. *Children's Assessment of Participation and Enjoyment & Preferences for Activities of Children (CAPE/PAC): User's Manual.* San Antonio, TX: Harcourt Assessment Inc; 2004.

37. Nagi S. Some conceptual issues in disability and rehabilitation. In: Sussman M, ed. *Sociology and Rehabilitation.* Washington, DC: American Sociological Association; 1965:100-113.

38. *Guide to Physical Therapist Practice.* Revised 2nd ed. Alexandria, VA: American Physical Therapy Association; 2003.

39. International Classification of Functioning, Disability and Health Web site. WHO, 2001, *Towards a Common Language for Functioning, Disability and Health,* http://www.who.int/classifications/icf/site/onlinebrowser/icf.cfm. Accessed October 12, 2006.

40. Rosenbaum P, Stewart D. The World Health Organization International Classification of Functioning, Disability, and Health: a model to guide clinical thinking, practice, and research in the field of cerebral palsy. *Semin Pediatr Neurol.* 2004;11:5-10.

41. Simeonsson RJ, Leonardi M, Lollar D, Bjrock-Akesson E, Hollenweger J, Martinuzzi A. Applying the International Classification of Functioning, Disability and Health (ICF) to measure childhood disability. *Disabil Rehabil.* 2003;25:602-610.

42. Law M, Baptiste S, Carswell A, McColl MA, Polatajko H, Pollock N. *Canadian Occupational Performance Measure.* 2nd ed. Toronto, Canada: Canadian Association of Occupational Therapists; 1994.

43. Missiuna C, Pollock N, Law M. *Perceived Efficacy and Goal Setting System. (PEGS).* San Antonio, TX: Psychological Corporation; 2004.

44. Missiuna C, Pollock N. Perceived efficacy and goal setting in young children. *Can J Occup Ther.* 2000;67:101-109.

45. Palisano RJ, Haley SM, Brown DA. Goal attainment scaling as a measure of change in infants with motor delays. *Phys Ther.* 1992;72:432-437.

46. Forbes DA. Goal Attainment Scaling. A responsive measure of client outcomes. *J Gerontol Nurs.* 1998;*24:34-40.*

47. Cusick A, McIntyre S, Novak I, Lannin N, Lowe K. A comparison of goal attainment scaling and the Canadian Occupational Performance Measure for paediatric rehabilitation research. *Pediatr Rehabil. 2006;9:149-157.*

48. Russell DJ, Rosenbaum PL, Cadman DT, Gowland C, Hardy S, Jarvis S. The Gross Motor Function Measure: a means to evaluate the effects of physical therapy. *Dev Med Child Neurol.* 1989;31:341-352.

49. Coster WJ, Deeney TM, Haltiwanger J, Haley SM. *School Function Assessment.* San Antonio, TX: The Psychological Corporation/Therapy Skill Builders; 1998.

50. Mancini MC, Coster WJ. Functional predictors of school participation by children with disabilities. *Occup Ther Int.* 2004;11:12-25.

51. Zabala J. The SETT framework: assistive technology training for appraisal personnel, handout #10. Houston, TX: Region IV Education Service Center; 1994.

5
Individualized Family Service Plans (IFSP)

Lynn Jeffries, PT, PhD, PCS

Requirements for every aspect of the development of an individualized family service plan (IFSP) are included in 34 CFR Section 303. The regulations cover evaluation and assessment; lead agency responsibilities; definition of early intervention services; general roles of service providers; time frames for IFSP development, implementation, and review; provisions for procedural safeguards; participants in and conduct of the IFSP meeting; service coordination; and provision of early intervention services. Family and professional collaboration and partnerships (see Chapter 2) in meeting these requirements are the keys to family-centered early intervention and to successful implementation of the IFSP process.

What is an IFSP?

According to Sec. 303.20:

> *Individualized family service plan or IFSP means a written plan for providing early intervention services to an infant or toddler with a disability under this part and the infant's or toddler's family.*

How does a child become eligible under Part C?

Infants and toddlers (and their families) are eligible for Part C services if the child meets the definition of "infant or toddler with a disability" as defined in Sec. 303.21 and in Chapter 3.

What are "early intervention services"?

Early intervention services, as described in Sec. 303.13(a) are:

> (1) *Are provided under public supervision;*
> (2) *Are selected in collaboration with the parents;*
> (3) *Are provided at no cost, except, subject to Secs. 303.520 and 303.521, where Federal or State law provides for a system of payments by families, including a schedule of sliding fees;*
> (4) *Are designed to meet the developmental needs of an infant or toddler with a disability and as requested by the family, the needs of the family to assist appropriately in the infant's or toddler's development, as identified by the individualized family service plan team, in any one or more of the following areas, including—*

(i) *Physical development;*
(ii) *Cognitive development;*
(iii) *Communication development;*
(iv) *Social or emotional development; or*
(v) *Adaptive development;*

(5) *Meet the standards of the State in which the services are provided, including the requirements of Part C of the Act;*
(6) *Include services identified under paragraph (b) of this section;*
(7) *Are provided by qualified personnel (as that term is defined in Sec. 303.31), including the types of personnel listed in paragraph (c) of this section;*
(8) *To the maximum extent appropriate, are provided in natural environments, as defined in Sec. 303.26 and consistent with Sec. 303.126; and*
(9) *Are provided in conformity with an individualized family service plan adopted in accordance with section 636 of the Act and Sec. 303.20.*

Who should be included in the IFSP meeting?

The IFSP meeting should include the parent(s) of the child, other family members if invited by the parents, an advocate if the parents request the presence of one, the service coordinator, person(s) involved in the evaluation and assessments, and the early intervention provider(s) who will be providing services for the child and family (Sec. 303.343[a]).

What are the requirements for an IFSP meeting?

Sec. 300.342(d) states:

(1) *IFSP meetings must be conducted—*
(i) *In settings and at times that are convenient to families;*
(ii) *In the native language of the family or other mode of communication used by the family, unless it is clearly not feasible to do so.*

(2) *Meeting arrangements must be made with, and written notice provided to, the family and other participants early enough before the meeting date to ensure that they will be able to attend.*

How soon after a child is referred to an early intervention program and determined to be eligible must the IFSP be written?

Within 45 days of the time the lead agency obtains parental consent to evaluate the child, the agency must appoint a service coordinator, complete the evaluation and assessment activities, and hold a meeting to develop the initial IFSP (Sec. 303.320[e] and 303.342[a]).

Do the regulations specify what must be included in the IFSP?

Yes. The content of the IFSP is outlined in Sec. 303.344. Although the regulations specify the information that must be included, the document is intended to be family-friendly and not simply an exercise in filling out paperwork. The IFSP must be developed with the full participation of the family and with service providers who truly believe that, given appropriate information, families know what is best for their children within the context of their own families.

Specifically, what must be included in the IFSP?

The general topics that must be addressed by the IFSP are listed in Sec. 303.344: information about the child's status, family information, results or outcomes, early intervention services to be provided, frequency and intensity of services, method of service delivery, other services to be provided, dates/duration of services, the name of the service coordinator, and the steps to be taken before the child transitions from Part C services.

What information about the child's status is required?

The IFSP must include a statement of the child's present levels of physical development (including motor development, vision, hearing, and health status), cognitive development, communication development, social or emotional development, and adaptive development, which includes self-help skills. This section must be based on information from the child's evaluation and assessment (Sec. 303.344[a]). Statements of levels of performance are more likely to be meaningful and of value to families if they are stated in terms of what the child can and cannot do as the child's performance relates to the family's concerns about the child, rather than providing scores on developmental tests.

What type of family information needs to be in the IFSP?

Family information is included only if the family agrees. A voluntary family assessment may help identify a family's resources and priorities.

> *With the concurrence of the family, the IFSP must include a statement of the family's resources, priorities, and concerns related to enhancing the development of the child (Sec. 303.344[b]).*

What is a voluntary family assessment?

A required part of the IFSP process is assessment of a family's needs, with the family's permission (Sec. 303.320[3][c]). A family assessment is a process that formally assists a family to identify their resources, priorities, and concerns, as well as the supports and services necessary for them to meet the developmental needs of their child. The assessment can be completed with an assessment tool or through interview. The family then decides how, when, and if they wish to use the information gained through the assessment process. If the family desires, the information gained through this process can become part of the child's IFSP. If a family assessment is carried out, the process should involve instruments that are sensitive to each family's ability to make its own decisions and the procedures implemented must provide families with multiple opportunities for expression of their concerns in both structured and open formats.[1,2]

How should the outcomes be written?

The family should identify the outcomes that they desire for their child and family. Family desired outcome statements are the driving force for the IFSP. Family-stated outcomes are generated by family members, members of the extended family, or individuals significant in the life of the child whose input the family desires. Outcomes usually are written in the IFSP document in a family's own words. Concerns of the other team members are introduced and included in the IFSP after all family concerns have been identified, and they are only included in the IFSP document with permission of the family and consensus of the team. Outcomes introduced by any team member should be written in jargon-free language that is understandable by the entire team. If team members disagree about appropriate outcomes, every effort must be made to reach a consensus, keeping in mind that the IFSP must reflect service needs and outcomes that represent the priorities of the family.[3-6]

What if a family does not identify outcomes or says, "You tell us, you're the expert"?

Families sometimes need assistance to identify appropriate outcomes. If families seem hesitant or unable to articulate their needs and desires for their child, team members should assist the family to identify them. Assisting families does not mean that service providers should suggest specific outcomes, but, through conversation and discussion, team members should ask questions about concerns the family may have during a typical day. Asking the family to describe a typical day can also provide insight into activities that may be difficult for them and their child.[7-10]

What should the outcome part of the IFSP include?

According to Sec. 303.344(c):

> *The IFSP must include a statement of the measurable results or measurable outcomes expected to be achieved for the child (including pre-literacy and language skills, as developmentally appropriate for the child) and family and the criteria, procedures and timelines that will be used to determine –*
> *The degree to which progress toward achieving the results of outcomes is being made; and*
> *Whether modifications of revisions of the results, outcomes, or services are necessary.*

The criteria for determining progress should relate to the intent of the outcome and the family's informed opinion about whether progress has occurred. This the most important measure of success.

How does a team write measurable outcomes based on the family's initial outcome statements?

Begin with the outcome the family has identified during the evaluation and assessment process and use this information in the development of the IFSP.[11-13] Families often say, for example, "I want my child to walk." During the development of the IFSP, the IFSP team could explore what "success" toward walking would look like for the family. Consider the family's typical routines when developing outcomes. Ask the question, "Would walking across the living room be considered success, or would walking with a walker from the living room to the kitchen be considered success?" Once the successful outcome is identified, the IFSP outcome statement can then be written in a measurable manner, such as: The child will use a reverse walker at home to go from the living room to the table for meals everyday for1week, by a set date.

Remember that each state's IFSP document includes the same information, but the formats are different. Some states begin with the family outcome, then have a statement of what progress will look like. This format allows the family's initial outcome in their own words to be identified and then the measurable statement included below it. Use the format your state requires, but remember that a measurable outcome must be identified so the team can determine the degree of progress toward achieving the outcome when it reviews the IFSP.

What is included in the IFSP section about early intervention services?

Sec 303.344(d), Early intervention services. says:

> *The IFSP must include a statement of the specific early intervention early intervention services, based on peer-reviewed research (to the extent practicable), that are necessary to meet the unique needs of the child and family to achieve the results or outcomes identified.*

In addition to stating who will provide what types of early intervention services, the IFSP also needs to describe the frequency, intensity, and method of delivering the services (Sec. 303.344[d][1][i][iii]). "Frequency and intensity" mean the number of days or sessions that a service will be provided, the length of time the service is provided during each session, and whether the service is provided on an individual or group basis (Sec. 303.344[d][2][i]). The "methods" mean how a service will be provided (Sec. 303.344[d][2][ii]).

What must be included in the duration of services section on the IFSP?

Dates and duration of services are covered under Sec. 303.344(f). The projected date for initiation of services must be listed on the IFSP. The date must be "as soon as possible" after the meeting for development of the IFSP. The duration of the services, or the ending date, must also be specified. The duration is a projection of when services will no longer be provided (such as when the child is expected to achieve the outcomes in the IFSP). If services are expected to continue until the IFSP is reviewed, then the review date would be the ending date.

How does the IFSP team identify services to meet the outcomes?

Part of identifying early intervention services is writing the strategies the early intervention providers and family will use to assist the child and family in meeting the IFSP outcomes. IFSP strategies document who will perform which routines, activities, and places to facilitate the achievement of the IFSP outcomes.[11]

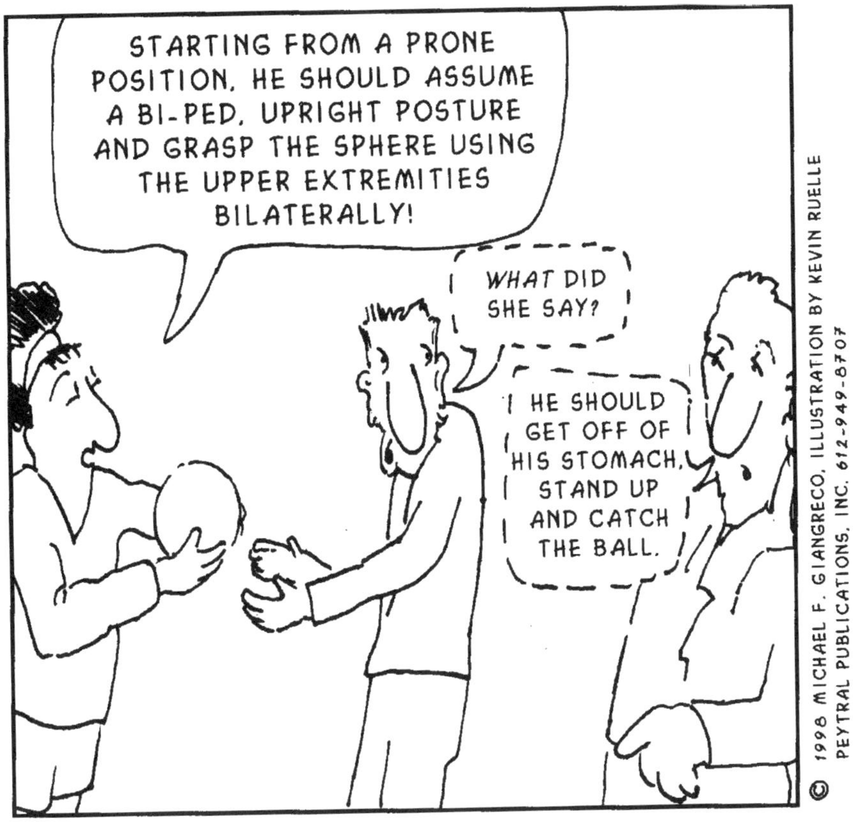
STARTING FROM A PRONE POSITION, HE SHOULD ASSUME A BI-PED, UPRIGHT POSTURE AND GRASP THE SPHERE USING THE UPPER EXTREMITIES BILATERALLY!
WHAT DID SHE SAY?
HE SHOULD GET OFF OF HIS STOMACH, STAND UP AND CATCH THE BALL.
© 1998 MICHAEL F. GIANGRECO, ILLUSTRATION BY KEVIN RUELLE
PEYTRAL PUBLICATIONS, INC. 612-949-8707

DAVID TRANSLATES FOR HANK WHO IS JUST LEARNING TO SPEAK JARGONESE AS A SECOND LANGUAGE.

A new requirement in IDEA 2004 is that early intervention services need to be based on peer-reviewed research, to the extent practicable, to meet the unique needs of the child and family. As team members develop the IFSP strategies, they should have a working knowledge of appropriate intervention strategies based on peer-reviewed research and use current best practice principles of family-centered services, provision of services in the child and family's natural environments, and consideration of the child and family's daily routines.[14-19]

Family-centered services means early intervention providers include the family in the decision-making and planning process as well as the intervention activities. As strategies are developed, the team considers the materials, toys, and equipment found within the child's home, the family's routines and activities, and the child and family's interests. The written strategies delineate who will do what to implement the plan, clearly identifying the activities without using professional jargon. (See Chapter 8 for more information about providing early intervention services in natural environments.)

How does the IFSP team provide the early intervention services?

A foundation of early intervention services is the inclusion of the child's family as part of the early intervention team. The most commonly used team models in early intervention are interdisciplinary and transdisciplinary models.[20] Although approaches may vary, typically when a team uses an interdisciplinary model, each team member performs separate assessments and identifies discipline-specific IFSP outcomes. Each interdisciplinary team member then works with the child and family during separate sessions and often focuses on intervention strategies specifically related to the provider's discipline. A speech pathologist, for example, would focus on the child's language development and the physical therapist would focus on the child's gross motor development. Team members then meet together to review the child's IFSP and discuss the child's progress with the other team members.

To facilitate communication and focus the child's and family's early intervention program, many early intervention teams use a transdisciplinary model of service delivery, in which a primary service provider is identified who can provide the services most relevant to the child's and family's needs at the current time.[20,21] The primary service provider then consults with and learns from other service providers to be able to provide a range of early intervention services that might not usually be associated with the primary service provider's own discipline. A physical therapist, for example, might be the primary service provider if a family's major concern is their child's motor development. If the outcomes also included communication and social skills, the physical therapist, in collaboration with other team members, such as a speech-language pathologist and child development specialist, would address communication and social skills in addition to motor skills.

In a transdisciplinary model of service delivery, all team members share the responsibility for success of the IFSP and for exchanging knowledge and skills with other team members. This model of service delivery is intended to result in greater integration of services than with an interdisciplinary model and reduces the need for children and families to cope with several service providers who may have a variety of opinions and recommendations.

Are assistive technology services and assistive technology devices early intervention services?

Yes. Sec. 303.13(1) describes assistive technology devices and services. The devices include:

> *... any item, piece of equipment or product system, whether acquired commercially off the shelf, modified, or customized, that is used to increase, maintain, or improve the functional capabilities of an infant of toddler with a disability. The term does not include a medical device that is surgically implanted, including cochlear implants, or the optimization (e.g., mapping) or the maintenance or replacement of that device.*

Assistive technology (AT) services include: the evaluation of the child's use of the device in the customary environment; the purchasing, leasing, or acquisition of the devices; the selecting, designing, fitting, customizing, adaptive, applying, maintaining, repairing, or replacing of the devices; the coordination of the therapy and intervention services; and the training of or provision of technical assistance to the child, family, and service provider working with the family (Sec. 303-13[1][ii]).

Physical therapists need to consider the child's need for AT. If the early intervention program has a specific AT team, it can be involved in AT services for the child. A service provider will need to initiate the involvement of the AT team and continue to support the child in the use of the AT devices once obtained. If the early intervention program does not have an AT team, then a service provider must evaluate the child's need for AT and provide the AT services identified on the IFSP, or identify an alternative source for AT evaluation and intervention. For more about assistive technology, refer to Chapter 10.

Does the IFSP need to state where services will be provided?

Yes. The location of services, including the natural environments in which services will be provided, must be specified (Sec. 303.344[d][ii-iii]).

What are considered to be "natural environments" in early intervention?

According to Sec. 303.26:

> *Settings that are natural or normal for an infant or toddler without a disability, may include the home.*

Services should not be provided in clinical settings or center-based early intervention programs simply because it is more convenient for service providers or because administrators will not permit service providers to go to the environments where the children are. When services are provided in other than the child's natural environment, it should be because that environment clearly most appropriately meets the needs of the child and the desires of the family. Providing physical therapy services in homes and other natural environments usually increases the likelihood that children will learn to use new skills in those settings, which is the goal of early intervention services. If services are provided in settings other than the natural environment, the IFSP team must justify in the IFSP the reasons for not providing services within a natural environment (Sec. 303.344[d][1][ii][B][1-3]). See Chapter 8 for more information about early intervention services in natural environments.

What are the "other services" that are included in the IFSP?

Other services include medical and any other services that the child and family needs or is receiving that are not required or funded through IDEA. Needed medical services, for example, which are not provided under Part C except for diagnostic purposes, might be included under "other services." For services not currently being provided, the IFSP must include a description of the steps the service coordinator or family will take to assist the child in obtaining the other services (Sec. 303.444[e]). The steps should include sources of funding that will pay for the services or describe how funds will be pursued.

What is a service coordinator?

Sec. 303.33 defines service coordination services as:

(a) Service coordination services means services provided by a service coordinator to assist and enable an infant or toddler with a disability and the child's family to receive the rights, procedural safeguards, and services that are authorized to be provided under Part C of the Act, including

(1) Coordinating all services required under this part across agency lines.

(2) Assisting parents of infants and toddlers with disabilities in gaining access to and coordinating the provision of early intervention services and coordinating other services identified in the IFSP under Sec. 303.344(e) that are needed or are being provided to the infant or toddler with a disability, and that child's family; and ....

The definition goes on to describe other activities of the service coordinator, the employment and assignment of service coordinators, and the qualifications of service coordinators (Sec. 303.33[b-c]).

What must be included within the IFSP regarding service coordination?

Sec. 303.344(g) says:

(1) The IFSP must include the name of the service coordinator from the profession most immediately relevant to the child's or families needs (or who is otherwise qualified to carry out all applicable responsibilities under this part), who will be responsible for the implementation of the early intervention services identified in a child's IFSP, including transition services, and coordination with other agencies and persons.

(2) In meeting the requirements in paragraph (g)(1) of this section, the term "profession" includes "service coordination."

Can a physical therapist be a service coordinator?

Whether a physical therapist can be a service coordinator depends on state regulations. Nothing in the federal law prohibits a physical therapist with knowledge of early intervention regulations and services from being a service coordinator. When a child's greatest needs are related to motor development, a physical therapist might be the most effective service coordinator.

What must the IFSP say about transition from Part C services?

Sec. 303.344(h)(1) the IFSP must include the steps to be taken to support the transition of the child to—

(i) Preschool services under Part B of the Act, to the extent that those services are appropriate;

(ii) Elementary school or preschool services (for children participating under Sec. 303.211);

(iii) Early education, Head Start and Early Head Start or child care programs; or

(iv) other appropriate services.

(2) The steps required in paragraph (h)(1) of this section include—

(i) Discussion with, and training of, parent, as appropriate, regarding future placements and other matters related to the child's transition;

(ii) Procedures to prepare the child for changes in service delivery, including steps to help the child adjust to, and function in, a new setting; and

The transmission of child find information about the child to the LEA or other relevant agency,

in accordance with Sec. 303.209(b) and, with parental consent, the transmission of information additional information to the LEA to ensure continuity of services, including evaluation and assessment information required in Sec. 303.320, and copies of IFSPs that have been developed and implemented in accordance with Sec. 303.340 through 303.345.
Identification of transition services and other activities that the IFSP team determine are necessary to support the transition of the child.

For more information about transition services, see Chapter 7.

How long should the IFSP be?

The IFSP does not need to be long and complicated. It should be family-friendly and useful as a working document for both the family and service providers. The IFSP should be clearly written and identify the services provided, actions to be taken to meet the IFSP outcomes, what the service coordinator will be doing, and what actions the family will be responsible for.

What are the requirements for parental consent?

During the IFSP meeting, the contents of the IFSP must be explained to the parents and they must give informed written consent before the early intervention services described in the plan are provided. If the parents do not consent to a part of the IFSP or withdraw consent to a part of the IFSP after giving it, those services cannot be provided. Services for which the parents give consent are provided (Sec. 303.342[e]).
If parents are fully involved in development of the IFSP, the IFSP is unlikely to include services that are unacceptable to them. Traditional roles of physical therapists and other service providers as experts who design and provide intervention for children and families are not acceptable for Part C programs. Rather, service providers provide open and honest opinions and express concerns based on their knowledge. Then families, as voluntary consumers of the services, choose their level of involvement, the roles they wish to assume, and the services they want to receive.

What is required for the periodic review of the IFSP?

Sec. 300.342(b) says:

(1) *A review of the IFSP for a child and the child's family must be conducted every six months or more frequently if conditions warrant, or if the family requests such a review. The purpose of the periodic review is to determine—*
  (i) *The degree to which progress toward achieving the outcomes is being made; and*
  (ii) *Whether modification or revision of the outcomes or services is necessary.*

The regulation goes on to say that the review can take place at a meeting, but could take place by another means if it is acceptable to the family and other people who need to participate in the review. Those who need to participate in the review include the parent(s), the service coordinator, and other family members, an advocate, or person outside of the family that the family wishes to attend. The regulation says people directly involved in conducting evaluations and assessments, and people providing services for the child and family must participate. If they are not able to attend the meeting, they may be involved through a telephone conference call, sending another knowledgeable representative, or making records available (Sec. 303.343[a-b]). When a child and family are receiving physical therapy services, then conditions probably warrant the physical therapist's participation in IFSP review.

What is an evaluation of the IFSP?

At least annually, a meeting must be held to determine if changes need to be made in the IFSP to meet the changing needs of the child and the child's family. Information from evaluations and ongoing assessment must be used to determine what services are needed and will be provided (Sec. 303.342[c]).

SUMMARY

The individualized family service plan (IFSP) is based on the family's desires for their child and the supports and services that the family needs to enhance their child's development. The IFSP document must include information about the child's status, family information (with the family's permission), outcomes, early intervention services to be provided, frequency and intensity of services, method of service delivery, other services to be provided, dates/duration of services, the name of the service coordinator, and the steps to be taken before the child transitions from Part C services.

REFERENCES

1. Bernheimer LP, Beogh BK. Weaving interventions into the fabric of everyday life: an approach to family assessment. *Top Early Child Special Educ.* 1995;15(4):415-433.
2. McGonigel M, Kaufmann R, Johnson B, eds. *Guidelines and Recommended Practices for the Individualized Family Service Plan.* 2nd ed. Bethesda, MD: Association for the Care of Children's Health; 1991.
3. Bailey DB. Collaborative goal-setting with families: resolving differences in values and priorities for services. *Top Early Child Special Educ.* 1987;7(2):59-71.
4. Brandt P. Negotiation and problem-solving strategies: collaboration between families and professionals. *Inf Young Child.* 1993;5(4):78-84.
5. McGonigel MJ, Garland CW. The individualized family service plan and the early intervention team: team and family issues and recommended practices. *Inf Young Child.* 1988;1(1):10-21.
6. Winton PJ. The family-focused interview: an assessment measure and goal-setting mechanism. In: Bailey DB, Simeonsson R, eds. *Family Assessment in Early Intervention.* Columbus, OH: Merrill; 1988:185-206.
7. Winton PJ, Bailey DB. Communicating with families: examining practices and facilitating change. In: Simeonsson JP, Simeonsson R, eds. *Understanding and Working With Parents of Children With Special Needs.* New York, NY: Holt, Rinehart, & Winston; 1993:210-230.
8. Cripe JW, Hanline MF, Daley SE. Preparing practitioners for planning intervention for natural environments. In: Winton PJ, McCollum JA, Catlett C, eds. *Reforming Personnel Preparation in Early Intervention: Issues, Models, and Practical Strategies.* Baltimore, MD: Paul H. Brookes; 1997:337-362.
9. Cripe JW, Venn ML. Family-guided routines for early intervention services. *Young Except Child.* 1997;1(1):18-26.
10. Wilson LL, Mott DW, Batman D. The asset-based context matrix: a tool for assessing children's learning opportunities and participation in natural environments. *Top Early Child Educ.* 2004;24(2):110-120.
11. Van Horn J, Gomm A, Davidman S. *New Mexico Infant Toddler Program: Technical Assistant Document. IFSPs.* Santa Fe, NM: New Mexico Department of Health, Longterm Care Division, Infant-Toddler Program; 2003.
12. Jung LA, Gomez C, Baird SM. Family-centered intervention: bridging the gap between IFSPs and implementation. In: Horn E, Ostrosky MM, Jones H, eds. *Family-Based Practices.* No. 5. *Young Except Children Monograph Series.* Longmont, CO: Sopris West Educational Services; 2003:61-76.
13. Jung LA, Grisham-Brown JL. Moving from assessment information to IFSPs: guidelines for the family-centered process. *Young Except Child.* 2006;9(2):2-11.
14. Trivette CM, Dunst CJ. DEC recommended practices: family-based practices. In: Sandall S, Hemmeter ML, Smith BJ, McLean ME, eds. *DEC Recommended Practices: A Comprehensive Guide for Practical Application in Early Intervention/Early Childhood Special Education.* Longmont, CO: Sopris West Educational Services; 2005:107-126.
15. McWilliam RA, Ferguson A, Harbin G, Porter DM, Vaderviere P. The family-centeredness of individualized family services plans. *Top Early Child Spec Educ.* 1998;18:69-82.
16. McWilliam RA. It's only natural…to have early intervention in the environments where it's needed. In: Sandall S, Ostrosky MM, eds. *Natural Environments and Inclusion.* No. 2. *Young Except Children Monograph Series.* Longmont, CO: Sopris West Educational Services; 2000:17-26.
17. Shelden ML, Rush DD. The ten myths about providing early intervention services in natural environments. *Inf Young Child.* 2002;14(1):1-13.
18. Bricker D, Pretti-Frontczak D, McComas N. *An Activity-Based Approach to Early Intervention.* 2nd ed. Baltimore, MD: Paul H. Brookes; 1998.
19. Pretti-Frontczak KL, Barr DM, Macy M, Cater A. Research and resources related to activity-based intervention, embedded learning opportunities and routines-based instruction. *Top Early Child Spec Educ.* 2003;23:29-39.
20. McWilliam RA. DEC recommended practices: interdisciplinary models. In: Sandall S, Hemmeter ML, Smith BJ, McLean ME, eds. *DEC Recommended Practices: A Comprehensive Guide for Practical Application in Early Intervention/Early Childhood Special Education.* Longmont, CO: Sopris West Educational Services; 2005:127-146.
21. McGonigel MJ, Woodruff G, Roszmann-Millican M. The transdisciplinary team: a model for family-centered early intervention. In: Johnson LJ, Gallagher RJ, LaMontagne MJ, et al, eds. *Meeting Early Intervention Challenges: Issues from Birth to Three.* 2nd ed. Baltimore, MD: Paul H. Brookes; 1994:95-131.

6
Individualized Education Programs (IEP)

Sandra Arnold, PT, PhD

Sections 300.320 through 300.325 of the federal regulations[1] include the requirements for every aspect of the IEP process, which is the set of procedures that govern how school districts should determine the educational services that a student requires.[1,2] The definition and content of the IEP are covered under Sec. 300.320. Regulations related to the IEP team, parental participation, development of the IEP, and other topics are covered in sections 300.321-300.325.

What is an IEP?

The individualized education program (IEP), which was introduced in Public Law (PL) 94-142, the Education for All Handicapped Children Act (EHA) of 1975, sets forth the free appropriate public education (FAPE) that is required for students with disabilities who are eligible to receive special education and related services under Part B of IDEA.[2] The IEP consists of 2 related parts: the IEP meeting and the IEP document. During the IEP meeting, the parents and school personnel collaborate to develop an educational program for the student (Sec. 300.320). Those attending the IEP meeting, as well as other individuals involved in developing the educational program for the student, are considered part of the IEP team. The federal regulations define the IEP document as "a written statement for a child with a disability that is developed, reviewed and revised in accordance with the provisions of IDEA" (Sec. 300.22).

How does a student become eligible to have an IEP?

Students who are eligible for special education and related services are eligible to have an IEP. Determining eligibility for special education and related services involves identification and evaluation processes that are covered in chapters 3 and 4. To briefly review, the evaluation process encompasses: (1) prior written consent of the parent; (2) a team that assesses the child in all areas related to the suspected disability; and (3) team decision-making to determine if the child has a disability as defined by IDEA, and if the child needs special education and related services (Sec. 300.304). Each state has forms used to document a student's evaluation, including a review of existing data, the evaluation results, and the team's summary and conclusions about the student.

How soon after the evaluation must the initial IEP be written?

The IEP team must meet within 30 calendar days after determining that a child requires special education and related services to develop a written IEP that documents the student's specific educational needs (Sec. 300.323[c][1]). Parents must be notified of the meeting in writing within sufficient time to attend the initial and subsequent IEP meetings. Note, however, that IDEA has no specific timetable for implementing the initial IEP. Section 300.323(c)(2) states as soon as possible following development of the initial IEP, special education and related services are made available to the child in accordance with the child's IEP. Subsequently, a student's IEP must be in effect at the beginning of each school year (Sec. 300.323[a]).

Who are the members of an IEP team?

Sec. 300.321(a) says the IEP team must include the following people:

(1) The parents of the child;
(2) Not less than one regular education teacher of the child (if the child is, or may be, participating in the regular education environment);
(3) Not less than one special education teacher of the child, or where appropriate, not less than one special education provider of the child;
(4) A representative of the public agency;
(5) An individual who can interpret the instructional implications of evaluation results, who may be a member of the team described in paragraphs (a)(2) through (6) of this section;
(6) At the discretion of the parent or the agency, other individuals who have knowledge or special expertise regarding the child, including related services personnel as appropriate; and
(7) Whenever appropriate, the child.

Must physical therapists attend IEP meetings?

Sec. 300.321(a)(6) says that the IEP team includes, at the discretion of the parent or the agency, other individuals who have knowledge or special expertise regarding the child, including related services personnel, as appropriate. Physical therapists should make every effort to attend IEP meetings for students who receive physical therapy or who might need physical therapy as a related service. Decisions about students' educational programs, including related services, are made at IEP meetings; therefore, the best time for physical therapists to provide input and hear the input of the rest of the team is during the meeting. Further, because IEP goals should be discipline-free and generated by the IEP team, physical therapists should not submit "physical therapy goals" before a meeting takes place. The only way a student's need for physical therapy and the goals of physical therapy can be determined is through the IEP process.

Sec. 300.321(e)(1) includes a provision for team members who can not attend IEP meetings:

> *A member of the IEP team is not required to attend an IEP Team meeting, in whole or in part, if the parent of a child with a disability and the public agency agree, in writing, that the attendance of the member is not necessary because the member's area of the curriculum or related services is not being modified or discussed at the meeting.*

Furthermore, Sec. 300.321(e)(2) states:

> *A member of the IEP Team may be excused from attending an IEP meeting, in whole or part, when the meeting involves a modification to or discussion of the member's area of the curriculum or related services, if—*
>
> *(i) The parent, in writing, and public agency consent to the excusal; and*
> *(ii) The member submits in writing to the parent and IEP Team, input into the development of the IEP prior to the meeting.*

What do you mean, "Never write physical therapy goals on an IEP"?

Writing "physical therapy goals" leads to physical therapy being an isolated service rather than a related service that directly enables a child to benefit from the educational program. A student's annual goals should be discipline-free; that is, the team decides which goals are most important for the student to accomplish, without regard to the discipline usually associated with them. The goals are the student's goals, not classroom goals, physical therapy goals, occupational therapy goals, and so on.[3] IDEA 2004 "does not require goals to be written for each specific discipline or to have outcomes and measures on a specific assessment tool"[1] (see Subpart G, "Analysis of Comments and Changes, Measurable Annual Goals" in the accompanying CD).

During the IEP meeting, the annual goals are determined by all team members. Then the people who will help the student achieve the goals are identified. Team members contribute to the development of the IEP by providing input from their own points of view and disciplinary perspectives to identify the most important and achievable goals for the student. These goals will and should vary with the student's age, abilities, and needs.

What if a physical therapist cannot attend the IEP meeting?

As described above, physical therapists are not required to attend IEP meetings if physical therapy services are not being modified or discussed, and if the parent and public agency consent to the absence in writing. However, physical therapsits should make every effort to attend each student's IEP meeting that will be addressing physical therapy services. If a physical therapist is unable to attend an IEP meeting due to illness or double-scheduled IEP meetings, he or she should consult with the student's teacher and parents prior to the meeting, to identify the strengths and concerns that are likely to be discussed during the IEP meeting. The physical therapist could then provide written information and suggestions related to those strengths and concerns. Physical therapists providing services under contract should attempt to include attending IEP meetings of the students on their caseloads within their contracts.

What is the role of parents in the IEP process?

Parents of a student with a disability are expected to be equal participants, along with school personnel, in developing, reviewing, and revising a child's IEP. The parents play an active role in discussions about the child's need for special education and related services, and join with school personnel in deciding what services the school district will provide to meet the child's needs.[4] This means that parents neither dictate the IEP, nor are they "out-voted" by school personnel. In fact, school personnel are obligated to encourage and support parents' participation by making them feel comfortable enough to contribute to the discussion, and by truly listening to their concerns and desires for their child. The focus of the IEP meeting should be to develop a plan that best addresses a student's strengths and needs—not just to fill out the paperwork correctly!

Where should the IEP meeting be held?

Parents must receive notification of the proposed time and place of the IEP meeting early enough to ensure that they will have an opportunity to attend (Sec. 300.322[a][1]). The time and place must be mutually agreeable to the parents and the rest of the IEP team (Sec. 300.322[a][2]). Customarily, the meeting is held during school hours, where the child attends school, in a comfortable room that encourages open communication of all team members.[5]

How should the IEP meeting be structured?

IDEA does not require a specific format for the IEP meeting.[2] The meeting must include the required participants and address the topics required under IDEA, and should adhere to the requirement that parents be treated as equal participants.[2]

Is the same written IEP form/document used in all states?

No, an "official" federal form does not exist and federal regulations do not mandate a format or specific length for the IEP document.[2] Each state has developed its own IEP format, which must include and adhere to all federal regulations relating to the IEP document and be understandable by parents.[2] Sometimes school districts develop their own state-approved IEP forms, thus each school district in a state may use a different form.

What components of the IEP are legally required?

In general, the IEP document is an individualized, legally binding commitment of resources that addresses the unique needs of the student. The IEP document must include the following components, listed under Sec. 300.320:

(a)(1) A statement of the child's present levels of academic achievement and functional performance, including—

(i) How the child's disability affects the child's involvement and progress in the general education curriculum (i.e., the same curriculum as for nondisabled children); or

(ii) For preschool children, as appropriate, how the disability affects the child's participation in appropriate activities;

(2) (i) A statement of measurable annual goals, including academic and functional goals designed to—

(A) Meet the child's needs that result from the child's disability to enable the child to be involved in and make progress in the general education curriculum; and

Meet each of the child's other educational needs that result from the child's disability;

(ii) For children with disabilities who take alternate assessments aligned to alternant achievement standards, a description of benchmarks or short-term objectives;

A description of –

(3) (i) How the child's progress toward meeting annual goals described in paragraph (2) of this section will be measured; and

When period reports on the progress the child is making toward meeting the annual goals (such as through the use of quarterly or other periodic reports, concurrent with the issuance of report cards) will be provided;

(4) A statement of the special education and related services and supplementary aids and services, based on peer-reviewed research to the extent practicable, to be provided to the child, or on behalf of the child, and a statement of the program modifications or supports for school personnel that will be provided for the child—

(i) To advance appropriately toward attaining the annual goals;

(ii) To be involved and make progress in the general education curriculum... and to participate in extracurricular and other nonacademic activities; and

(iii) To be educated and participate with other children with disabilities and nondisabled children in the activities described in this section;

(5) An explanation of the extent, if any, to which the child will not participate with nondisabled children in the regular class and in the activities describe in this section;

(6) (i) A statement of any individual appropriate accommodations that are necessary to measure the academic achievement and functional performance of the child on State or district-wide assessments ... and

(ii) If the IEP Team determines that the child must take an alternate assessment instead of a particular regular State or district wide assessment of student achievement, a statement of why—

(A) The child cannot participate in the regular assessment; and

(B) The particular alternate assessment selected is appropriate for the child; and

(7) The projected date for the beginning of the services and modifications, and the anticipated frequency, location, and duration of those services and modifications.

(b) Transition Services. Beginning not later than the first IEP to be in effect when the child turns 16, or younger if determined appropriate by the IEP Team, and updated annually, thereafter, the IEP must include-

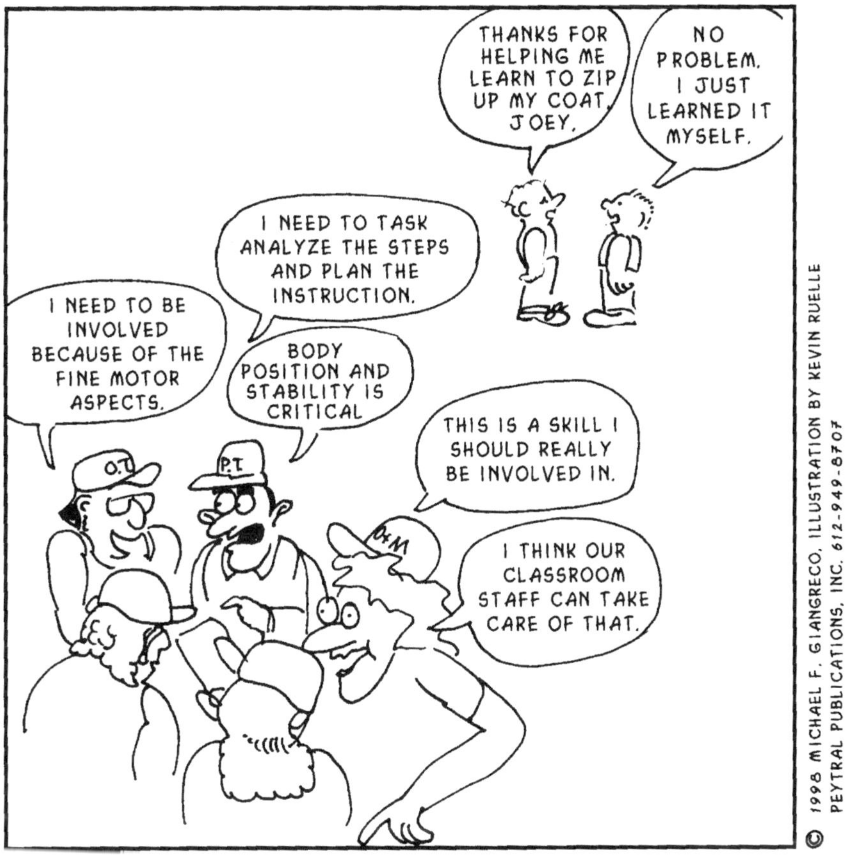
THANKS FOR HELPING ME LEARN TO ZIP UP MY COAT, JOEY.
NO PROBLEM. I JUST LEARNED IT MYSELF.
I NEED TO TASK ANALYZE THE STEPS AND PLAN THE INSTRUCTION.
I NEED TO BE INVOLVED BECAUSE OF THE FINE MOTOR ASPECTS.
BODY POSITION AND STABILITY IS CRITICAL
THIS IS A SKILL I SHOULD REALLY BE INVOLVED IN.
I THINK OUR CLASSROOM STAFF CAN TAKE CARE OF THAT.
O.T.
P.T.
O+M
© 1998 MICHAEL F. GIANGRECO, ILLUSTRATION BY KEVIN RUELLE
PEYTRAL PUBLICATIONS, INC. 612-949-8707

ADVENTURES IN ZIPPING

ZONE OF PROXIMAL CONFUSION

> (1) *Appropriate measurable postsecondary goals based upon age appropriate transition assessments related to training, education, employment, and where appropriate, independent living skills; and The transition services (including courses of study) needed to assist the child in reaching those goals.*
>
> (c) *Transfer of rights at age of majority. Beginning not later than one year before the child reaches the age of majority under State law, the IEP must include a statement that the child has been informed of the child's rights under Part B of the Act, if any, that will transfer to the child on reaching the age of majority.*

States may determine the extent to which they use short-term objectives and benchmarks in the IEP[1] (see Subpart G, "Analysis of Comments and Changes, Measurable Annual Goals" on the accompanying CD). If a state requires benchmarks or short-term objectives, the state must identify in writing to the LEA its policy, which is not required by Part B of IDEA 2004 or the federal regulations.[1]

What should be included under statement of the child's present levels of academic achievement and functional performance?

This section of the IEP describes the disability-related concerns that interfere with the student's achievement and performance so that meaningful goals can be developed. This information provides a baseline for designing and measuring the students' annual goals. Although the terms *academic achievement* and *functional performance* are not defined in the federal regulations, they are presumed to mean the child's current, unique performance in academic areas, and in participation in the general curriculum, including nonacademic areas.[2] The general education curriculum, means "the same curriculum as for nondisabled children" (Sec. 300.320[a][1][i]). The student information is gathered from a variety of sources including evaluation and statewide assessment results, and observations and interviews from the parent, teacher, and related service personnel.

Physical therapists participate with the IEP team in writing statements on the IEP about the student's present levels of academic achievement and functional performance.

What should annual goals address?

Measurable annual goals are critical to the planning process used to develop and implement the IEP. Once the IEP team has developed measurable annual goals for a student, the team can develop strategies that will be most effective to help the student achieve those goals. In addition to being discipline-free, as previously described, annual goals should be functional, chronologically age-appropriate, and meaningful to the student and the student's family. Goals should also include activities that the student can perform frequently and should address both the present and the future needs of the student, including a vision toward postsecondary life.[6]

What is a functional goal?

A useful definition of a *functional goal* is an activity that must be done by another person if the student does not do it.[7] Obviously, a wide variety of activities are functional and the selected goals will depend on a student's abilities and many other factors, such as the possibility of the student keeping up with a general education curriculum and the family's desires. Getting to class on time, eating lunch independently, playing safely on the playground, writing one's name on class work, deciding which book to read during free reading time, and successful completion of college ACT tests with appropriate modifications are just a few functional activities that might become annual goals.

"Functional" also means that the student will be active; that is, the student will do something.[8] Goals include the word "will," such as the student will get his own lunch or the student will achieve a certain level in math. It is important to differentiate things that people will do for the student, such as acquire a wheelchair, from things the student will learn to do. Things that other people do are not written into the IEP as goals. They are written as services to be provided. It also is important to avoid making goals of passive activities the student does, such as "tolerate" standing. Instead, state the active behavior the student will accomplish or write the activity as a service to be provided, such as positioning.

How can goals be chronologically age-appropriate when a student functions at a much lower level developmentally?

Students should be engaged in activities in which peers of the same age would participate. It would be inappropriate, for example, for a 9-year-old boy with severe cognitive and motor delays to be playing with a baby doll or a busy box on a mat on the floor. If the goals for the student addressed both independent play and making choices, perhaps a soft baseball or a super-hero toy could replace the baby doll and a tape recorder with the student's favorite songs, radio, or computer with switch access could replace the busy box. Also, most students should be upright, rather than lying on the floor, when engaging in school activities. Physical therapists and other service providers must be creative to develop age-appropriate activities, particularly for students with severe disabilities, especially as the student approaches adulthood. Some classic sources by Giangreco, Cloninger, and Iverson,[9] Rainforth and York,[10] and York and Vandercook[11] provide useful information about the importance of age-appropriate activities and some creative suggestions for identifying them.

What are meaningful goals that are used frequently across a variety of environments?

Meaningful goals are goals that the child, the parents, and other IEP team members think are particularly important for the student to learn. They are also based on expectations for what the child will do when becoming an adult. A family, for example, may think that independent toileting by the student would make a big difference in the lives of both the family and the student. Some of the goals that physical therapists used to write were not meaningful to families, students, or other team members—such as propping while in the prone position on a wedge, standing on one foot, maintaining the half-kneeling position, and similar developmental skills. Although the importance of practicing such skills is debatable, particularly for school-age children,[12-14] the activity should result in accomplishment of a meaningful goal, such as walking up the stairs to reach a classroom or job or to participate in activities on a stage.

When activities are used frequently across a variety of environments, students have many opportunities to learn. Students are in school for only a small part of their lives; therefore, educational goals need to address tasks/activities that students likely will perform often on a daily basis. The tasks should also be used in the future in a variety of environments. If a physical therapist works with a student to squat, pick up a beanbag, and then stand to throw the beanbag in a bucket, but the student has no opportunities to practice similar activities outside of the therapy session, the benefit of the activity is questionable. Similarly, working on a more functional activity, such as getting a drink from a particular drinking fountain, is unlikely to be either important or learned unless the student has many opportunities to drink from similar drinking fountains. Some examples of frequently used activities that are used across a variety of environments include: drinking from a straw, unbuckling a seat belt, transferring to a toilet, using a computer, writing one's name (either with a pencil or with a word processor), and communicating effectively.

What kind of goals meet present and/or future needs?

Students with disabilities often take a long time to learn a few things.[15] It is important, therefore, to select goals that not only will meet present needs, but will meet the student's needs in the future. We cannot assume that by working on "prerequisite" skills that students will eventually accomplish skills needed in the future. Example of goals that probably will not meet future needs are developmental activities that are rarely used by adults, such as walking on a balance beam, using play money, and naming pictures. Some goals that could help to meet future needs include independent mobility, bearing weight to assist with transfers, and learning to use assistive technology devices for functional purposes.

How do teams write functional, discipline-free, chronologically age-appropriate, meaningful goals?

Student goals are not difficult to write if the IEP team has a clear understanding of the strengths and needs of the student. Because the goals are the student's, and not the physical therapist's, they are derived by the desires and needs of the student. Student goals should not be confused with intervention plans. Through the IEP process, for example, a team may discover that Jose, a seventh-grader with cerebral palsy, Gross Motor Function Classification System (GMFCS)[16] Level III, does not want to be late for his first-hour class, but is having difficulty navigating the hallways after the first-hour bell. A functional, discipline-free, chronologically age-appropriate, meaningful goal might be, "Jose will walk with his walker from his homeroom to his first-hour class in the time required by his peers 3 out of 4 mornings each week by November 30." This is a measurable goal that is meaningful to Jose. A physical therapy intervention plan to assist with obtaining this goal might include working on impairments that the PT believes are limiting his walking, such as walking a particular distance, balance or stride length, or improving timing, but these are not the actual functional goal. Improving impairments may not lead to improved walking and also is not likely to be of interest to Jose, who wants to keep up with his peers and not be late to class. Although intervention plans may include activities to improve impairments, they should also include actual practice of the functional skill; for example, walking in the hall during passing time. Other examples of goals are:

1. Jenny will climb the ladder of the "big" playground slide and slide down independently with her peers 2 times each day for 5 consecutive outside recess school days by March 31.
2. Shane will carry his lunch tray from the lunch line to the lunch table, without spilling his milk or food, every day at lunch for 10 consecutive school days by May 30.
3. After story time, Jasmine will stand up from her carpet square, using the bookshelf for support, when the teacher says, "Our story is over, it's time for table work," 3 times per week for1month by May 31.

Goals also are based on the best available evidence. In determining student goals, the IEP team members choose goals they think the student can accomplish in1year. Prognostic information related the student's disability is helpful in determining appropriate goals. In the above example, if Jose's classification on the GMFCS were Level IV, goals related to walking with a walker in a busy hallway would need to be seriously considered.[17] Current evidence suggests that children classified at Level IV are not likely to walk long distances with a walker.[17]

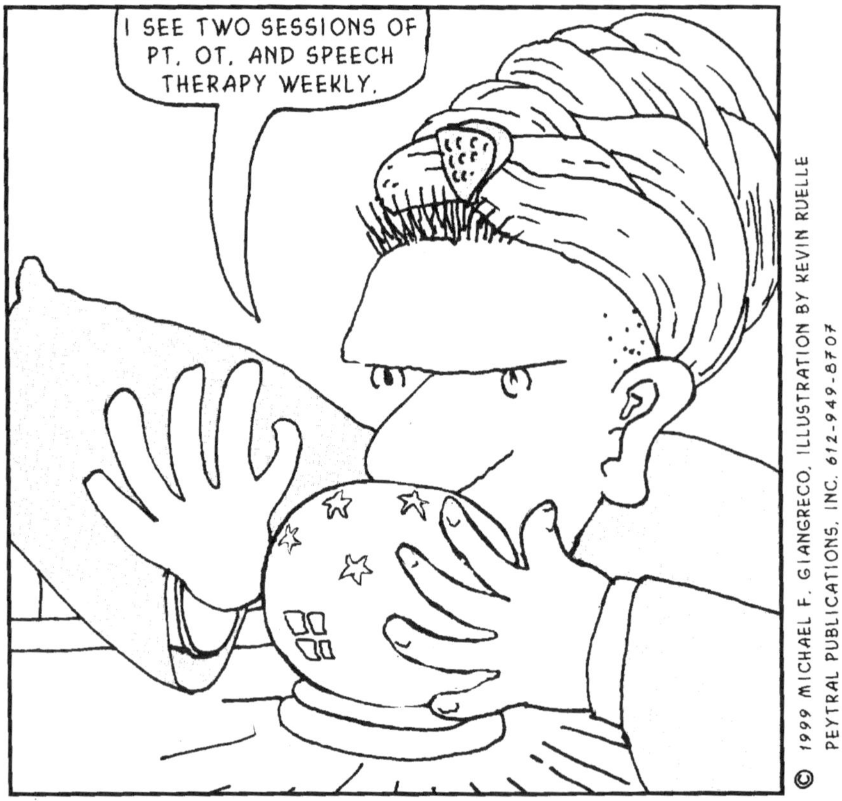

THE DISTRICT'S EXPERIMENTAL METHOD FOR DETERMINING RELATED SERVICES WORKS JUST AS WELL AS MAKING THOSE DECISIONS BEFORE KNOWING A STUDENT'S IEP GOALS AND OTHER LEARNING OUTCOMES.

Who decides if physical therapy should be included in the IEP?

The IEP team decides if physical therapy services "are required to assist a child with a disability to benefit from special education" (Sec. 300.34[a]). The team first identifies the educational goals and objectives, and later makes a placement decision. After the placement decisions have been made, the team then decides which professionals are needed to assist the student to achieve educational goals, or to have access to and participate in the educational environment. Related services decisions are made based on which, if any, related services the student needs. Note that neither physical therapy nor other services should be determined by a student's scores on a test; decisions must be based on students' unique needs, including those of teachers and others in the student's environment who might need to learn to assist the child (see Chapter 3).

Although a student may have disability that might require physical therapy, the student may not need school-based physical therapy services because the student does not need them to benefit from special education. It is OK for a student with a disability to *not* receive physical therapy services if the team determines that student's goals do not require the expertise of a physical therapist for the student to attain them. As an example, an 8-year-old student with spina bifida who is independently mobile on the school campus in her custom wheelchair may not need physical therapy services, particularly if the student's goals are related to reading comprehension, staying on task, and writing.

May parents stipulate the amount of therapy a student will receive?

Parents certainly may make a recommendation. It is not appropriate for parents or other team members, however, to make recommendations based solely on the child's diagnosis or disability, or without considering the capabilities of the rest of the team to help the child to achieve the identified goals. A more appropriate approach is to focus on the outcomes desired for the child (the goals), determine the type of expertise needed to help the child achieve those outcomes, and then determine who on the team has that expertise and how much time will be required.[18] If the desired outcome for a child is to walk to the cafeteria, for example, the team may need guidance from the physical therapist. Depending on the knowledge and skills of other team members, that guidance may be 5 times per week or only 1 time per month. It also may be that an occupational therapist who already works with the child can address this need, or that the child's special education teacher has the necessary knowledge and skill and does not need support from a related service provider.

Must the amount of physical therapy services be documented on the IEP?

Yes. The amount of physical therapy services that will be provided must be written on the IEP so that all team members will have a clear understanding of the level of commitment of resources to be provided by the school district.[1,2] The US Department of Education's Office of Special Education Programs (OSEP) has stated, however, that school districts are not required to specify the amount of services to be provided in terms of hours and minutes to comply with IDEA. [2] Rather, "the amount of time to be committed to each of the various services to be provided must be appropriate to the specific service, and clearly stated in the IEP in a manner that can be understood by all involved in the development and implementation of the IEP"[1] (see Subpart G, "Analysis of Comments and Changes, Initiation, Frequency, Location, and Duration of Services," on the CD with this book). As answered in question 35 in the Appendix of 34 CFR 300 for IDEA 1997,[19] the amount of special education or related service to be provided to a child may be stated on the IEP as a range (eg, physical therapy to be provided 3 times per week for 30-45 minutes per session) only if the IEP team determines that stating the amount of services as a range is necessary to meet the unique needs of the child. A range may not be used because of personnel shortages or uncertainty regarding the availability of staff.

The frequency statement should not lock therapists into providing services only on a specific day of the week (eg, only on Thursday mornings at 10:00 am). The amount of time specified on the IEP should include not only contact with the child, but all activities that directly relate to that child, such as making phone calls to vendors and doctors, attending IEP meetings, working with the child's assistive technology in relevant environments, and consulting with teachers, parents, and other people involved in helping students meet their educational goals.

When are placement decisions made?

The IEP team makes decisions about the location(s) in which a student will receive special education and related services based on the student's completed IEP, considering the most appropriate educational services and environment for the student (Sec. 300.116). The team's placement decisions reflect the student's previously established educational goals and unique needs. In the past, IEP teams often placed students in programs or classrooms based on their disability categories, rather than identifying the least restrictive environment in which the child's IEP could be carried out with the necessary supports. Each child's placement decision also:

(a) (1) Is made by a group of persons, including the parents, and other persons knowledgeable about the child, the meaning of the evaluation data, and the placement options

(2) Is made in conformity with the LRE provisions of this subpart.

(b) (1) Is determined at least annually;

(2) Is based on the child's IEP: and

(3) Is as close as possible to the child's home;

(c) Unless the IEP of a child requires some other arrangement, the child is educated in the school that he or she would attend if nondisabled;

> (d) *In selecting the LRE (least restrictive environment), consideration is given to any potential harmful effect on the child or on the quality of services that he or she needs; and*
> (e) *A child with a disability is not removed from education in age-appropriate regular classrooms solely because of needed modifications in the general curriculum. (Sec. 300.116)*

A continuum of alternative placements must be available. These may include, for example, regular classes full time, special classes part time, special classes full time, instruction at home, in the hospital, or in other settings (Sec. 300.115[b][1]). Students with disabilities must be educated with peers without disabilities to the maximum extent possible, and they may be removed from the regular educational environment only when the "nature or severity of the disability is such that education in regular classes with the use of supplementary aids and services cannot be achieved satisfactorily" (Sec. 300.114[a][2]).

What are supplementary aids and services?

Sec. 300.42 Supplementary aids and services says:

> *... aids and services means aids, services, and other supports that are provided in regular education classes or other education-related settings and in extracurricular and nonacademic settings, to enable children with disabilities to be educated with nondisabled children to the maximum extent appropriate in accordance with Secs. 300.114-300.116.*

Supplementary aids and services may include modification of how information is presented and how the student is expected to perform or respond; adjustments of time and quantity of work; alternative materials and classroom equipment; behavior interventions; assistive technology devices and services; and other innovative approaches in the regular classroom that will enable the child to participate and learn in the general education environment. Some other examples of supplementary aids and services are training for a teacher (Sec. 300.119); student support from a paraprofessional, co-teacher, or related service provider in the classroom[9]; assistive technology devices or services to enable a student to participate in a vocational training program in the community; or training for a job coach who is working with a student to assess vocational options after high school.

Can physical therapists change the goals or frequency of physical therapy on an IEP during the school year?

The IEP must be in place at the beginning of each school year and must be reviewed periodically, but at least annually (300.324[b][1][i]). The IEP team may, however, review it more frequently, at which time the team may change goals, objectives, frequency, and other IEP elements. In making changes to a student's IEP, the parent and the public agency may agree not to convene the IEP team and instead may develop a written document to amend or modify the student's current IEP, and ensure that the IEP team is informed of the changes (300.324[4]).

SUMMARY

The IEP is a process that includes both the IEP team meeting and writing the IEP document. IEP teams collaboratively develop individualized goals for students with disabilities receiving special education and related services. Parents, and students when appropriate, always are a part of the team. Physical therapists are considered part of the IEP team as "individuals who have knowledge or special expertise regarding the child," as specified in IDEA. The role of a physical therapist is not to develop "PT goals," but rather to participate in the collaborative development of students' educational goals along with the other members of IEP teams.

REFERENCES

1. 34 CFR Part 300 (2006).
2. Norlin JW. *What Do I Do When...The Answer Book on Individualized Education Programs.* 3rd ed. Horsham, PA: LPR Publications; 2007.
3. Bundy AC. Assessment and intervention in school-based practice: answering questions and minimizing discrepancies. In: McEwen IR, ed. *Occupational and Physical Therapy in Educational Environments.* Binghamton, NY: Haworth Press; 1995:69-88.

4. Turnbull AP, Turnbull HR. *Families, Professionals, and Exceptity: A Special Partnership.* 2nd ed. Upper Saddle River, NJ: Prentice-Hall; 1997.
5. Bateman B. *Better IEPs.* Cresswell, OR: Otter Ink; 1995.
6. Rainforth B, York-Barr J. *Collaborative Teams for Students with Severe Disabilities: Integrating Therapy and Educational Services.* 2nd ed. Baltimore, MD: Paul H. Brookes; 1997.
7. Brown L, Branston MB, Hamre-Nietupski S, Pumpian I, Certo N, Gruenewald L. A strategy for developing chronological age appropriate and functional curriculum content for severely handicapped adolescents and young adults. *J Special Ed.* 1979;12:81-90.
8. Downing J. Active versus passive programming: a critique of IEP objectives for students with the most severe disabilities. *J Assoc Sev Handicap.* 1988;13:197-201.
9. Giangreco MF, Cloninger CJ, Iverson VS. *Choosing Options and Accommodations for Children: A Guide to Educational Planning for Students with Disabilities.* 2nd ed. Baltimore, MD: Paul H. Brookes Publishing; 1993.
10. Rainforth B, York J. Integrating related services in community instruction. *J Assoc Sev Handicap.* 1987;12:190-198.
11. York J, Vandercook T. Designing an integrated program for learners with severe disabilities. *Teaching Except Children.* 1991;Winter:22-28.
12. Atwater S. Should the normal developmental sequence be used as a theoretical model in pediatric physical therapy? In: Lister MJ, ed. *Contemporary Management of Motor Control Problems: Proceedings of the II STEP Conference.* Alexandria, VaA Foundation for Physical Therapy: 1991:89-93.
13. Harris S. Functional abilities in context. In: Lister MJ, ed. *Contemporary Management of Motor Control Problems: Proceedings of the II STEP Conference.* Alexandria, VA: Foundation for Physical Therapy: 1991:253-259.
14. McEwen IR, Shelden ML. Pediatric therapy in the 1990s: the demise of the educational versus medical dichotomy. In: McEwen IR, ed. *Occupational and Physical Therapy in Educational Environments.* New York, NY: Haworth Press; 1995:33-45.
15. Brown L, Long E, Udvari-Solner A, et al. Should students with severe intellectual disabilities be based in regular or in special education classrooms in home schools? *J Assoc Sev Handicap.* 1989;14:8-12.
16. Palisano R, Rosenbaum P, Walter S, Russell D, Wood E, Galuppi B. Development and reliability of a system to classify gross motor function in children with cerebral palsy. *Dev Med Child Neurol.* 1997;39:214-223.
17. Palisano RJ, Hanna SE, Rosenbaum PI, et al. Validation of a model of gross motor function for children with cerebral palsy. *Phys Ther.* 2000;80:974-983.
18. Giangreco MF. *Vermont Interdependent Services Team Approach: A Guide to Coordinating Educational Support Services.* Baltimore, MD: Paul H. Brookes; 1996.
19. 34 CFR Part 300 (1999).

7 Transition

Julie Smith, MS, OTR/L and Lorraine Sylvester, PT, MS

Transition is change—change from 1 status to another. Children with disabilities and their families experience many transitions throughout life, such as from home to preschool, to elementary and middle school, to high school, and eventually to adulthood. For young children receiving early intervention services under IDEA, transition is a set of activities that occur 3 to 9 months prior to a child's third birthday to prepare the child to graduate from Part C services (Sec. 300.124, 303.209). As children receiving services under Part B approach adolescence and adulthood, transition also describes the activities that must occur no later than age 16 to prepare students to move from high school to postsecondary activities (Sec. 300.43).

What does transition from early intervention (Part C) at age 3 involve?

Transition from Part C involves step-by-step procedures to support a child's smooth and effective transition from early intervention services at age 3 to preschool, school, or other appropriate services or to leave the early intervention program without need for further specialized services (Sec. 303.209, 300.124). The early intervention team must develop and document a transition plan on the individualized family service plan (IFSP) for each child a minimum of 90 days and not more than 9 months before the child's third birthday. IDEA requires documentation of 4 steps to address activities and services that the child and family need for transition.

First Step

The first step entails "discussion with, and training of, parents, as appropriate, regarding future placements and other matters related to the child's transition" (Sec. 303.344[h][2][i]). Strategies to help parents learn about and participate in transition include (1) parent education workshops and individual support,[1-2] (2) parent-to-parent programs,[3] and (3) identifying parent preferences about involvement and information needs.[1-3]

Families have reported satisfaction with parent education workshops on such topics as: (1) what transition means and includes, (2) team member roles, (3) matching the needs of the child and programs, (4) program options and services, (5) effective communication, (6) the law and educational rights, (7) preparation of the child, and (8) participation in the individualized education program (IEP) meeting.[2,4] Individual supports to families include collaborative activities such as developing transition plans, visiting programs, identifying timelines with required and recommended activities, making referrals, assisting with strategies to share information with other programs, and preparing for an IEP meeting.[1-2]

Parent-to-parent programs are another way to help families. These programs offer parents an opportunity to learn from others who have already been through transition[3] and to get a perspective from outside the service systems.

To help service personnel identify parent preferences about involvement in the transition process and information needs, several authors described checklists and sample questions.[1,3] The level of involvement differs from 1 family to another. Some questions about a parent's desired level of involvement include: (1) Would you like help developing goals that will prepare your child for transition?, (2) Would you like to talk with other parents who have transitioned from our program?, and (3) Would you like to visit with staff from other programs?

The method of learning about transition also differs from 1 parent to another. Rous, Hemmeter, and Schuster[5] recommend that service personnel provide information in a manner that matches the parent's learning style. Information provided to families might include written materials, individual assistance, group instruction, electronic materials (DVD, videotape, or audiotape), or visiting programs.

When discussing future placement options with parents, careful consideration of an appropriate environment for meeting the educational needs of a child at age 3 is essential. The environment must be selected from a variety of options, be the least restrictive environment (LRE) for the child, and be as close to the child's home as possible. The service site options for preschool children must include, but not be limited to, public and private preschools, other community programs, and the child's home.

Second Step

The second transition step to document on the IFSP involves "procedures to prepare the child for changes in service delivery, including steps to help the child adjust to, and function in, a new setting" (Sec. 303.344[h][2][ii]). A child's success when moving from 1 program to another depends on the child's ability to cope and the activities provided to prepare the child for change.[3] Early intervention personnel knowledgeable about strategies that reduce stress and teach coping skills and routines to support the child in the LRE increase the likelihood of success.[2] Rosenkoetter et al[3] described 6 strategies to prepare children for future changes: (1) help the child anticipate the change by answering questions and commenting positively about new staff, the environment, and activities; (2) read books about transition; (3) role play routines and meeting new staff and children; (4) visit programs when other children are and are not present; (5) make any necessary changes in sleep and meal routines; (6) encourage and develop positive relationships with new service personnel as a gradual separation from early intervention staff occur; and (7) teach targeted developmentally appropriate skills and routines for a new environment.

For children who will receive services in an early childhood setting, an understanding of preschool entry-level skills and methods to assess skills are necessary to adequately prepare children for a change in services.[2,3,5] The Helpful Entry Level Skills Checklist (HELS)[6,7] and the Hawaii Preparing for Integrated Preschool (PIP) Assessment[2,8] are tools that address critical skills for preschool environments. The HELS is a screening tool used to determine a child's needs in the areas of social, behavioral, and functional skills. Included are classroom rules, work skills, communication, social behavior (eg, cooperation, turn taking, and sharing), and self-management. The PIP identifies 30 survival skills preschool teachers said are critical for success for children 3 years of age. Skills most expected include appropriate classroom behavior, social/play skills, and self-care.[8] Rosenkoetter et al[3] provide a list of social, communication, adaptive, and cognitive skills that aid transition to preschool. The authors caution service personnel, however, not to use the skills as prerequisites or criteria for inclusion in a preschool program.

Third Step

The third transition step to document on the IFSP involves transmitting information to the local education agency (LEA). According to Sec. 303.344(h)(2)(iii), the early intervention program is required to provide child find information in accordance with Sec. 303.209(b). With parental permission, the early intervention program may transmit additional information including evaluations, assessments, and copies of the IFSP.

The transmission of information also involves preparing families to share information about their children, their desires for their children, and how they want to be involved in services with the receiving programs. Families should be encouraged to identify their preferred method of giving information. Child portfolios, videos, photographs, and formal or informal discussions are a few examples. Hains et al[1] outlined a guide to help families share information with receiving programs. The guide includes information about the child, family involvement, preferred communication method with the receiving program staff, and questions the family wants to ask.

IDEA requires early intervention personnel to schedule and facilitate a transition planning conference with the family, LEA, and community programs, with parental consent (Sec. 303.209[c][1-2]). The transition planning conference provides families a venue to share information, learn more specifically about services that receiving programs offer, learn whether more and what information is needed to determine eligibility for the programs, and to further define activities and timelines for a "smooth and effective" transition. The transition planning conference is to occur a minimum of 90 days and not more than 9 months prior to the child's third birthday. The LEA is required to participate in the transition planning conference (Sec. 300.124[c]).

Fourth Step

The fourth step to document on the IFSP includes "identification of transition services and other activities that the IFSP team determines are necessary to support the transition of the child" (Sec. 303.344[h][iv]). The team considers additional activities to ensure a smooth and effective transition. Examples of activities include collaborating with receiving program staff to complete an evaluation to determine eligibility, training teachers and other personnel in the use of assistive technology, or sharing effective behavioral strategies with new program staff.

When a child transitions from Part C to Part B, does the child have to be retested for eligibility?

Within the requirements on IDEA, each state has determined its own eligibility criteria for Part C and Part B. In states that have different eligibility requirements for Part C and Part B, eligibility for the receiving program must be determined as the child approaches age 3. Ideally, sending and receiving programs and agencies work closely together to prevent redundancy in evaluations and, with permission from the family, share appropriate information for determining eligibility for programs. Collaboration between programs assists in reducing gaps in services.

What does transition from early intervention (Part C) involve for states that have elected to provide early intervention services to children ages 3 and older?

States may choose to continue to provide early intervention services for children ages 3 and older until they enter kindergarten or elementary school (Sec. 303.211). The children must have received early intervention services prior to the age of 3, and they must meet eligibility requirements under Section 619 of Part B. States may choose to serve all children with disabilities ages 3 through 5, or 1 of 3 subsets. According to Sec. 303.211(a)(2)(i-iii):

> (2) *A State that adopts the policy described in paragraph (a)(1) of this section may determine whether it applies to children with disabilities ages three through five inclusive, or to one of the following three subsets of that age range:*
> (i) *From age three until the beginning of the school year following the child's third birthday.*
> (ii) *From age three until the beginning of the school year following the child's fourth birthday.*
> (iii) *From age three until the beginning of the school year following the child's fifth birthday.*

States that choose the option to make early intervention services available to children ages 3 and older must meet several requirements. According to Sec. 303.211(b)(1-7):

> (b) *Requirements. If a State's application for a grant under this part includes the State policy described in paragraph (a) of this section, the system must ensure the following:*
> (1) *Parents of children with disabilities served pursuant to this section are provided annual notice that contains—*
> (i) *A description of the rights of the parents to elect to receive services pursuant to this section or under Part B of the Act; and*

(ii) An explanation of the differences between services provided pursuant to this section and services provided under Part B of the Act, including—

(A) The types of services and the locations at which the services are provided;

(B) The procedural safeguards that apply; and

(C) Possible costs (including the costs or fees to be charged to families as described in Sec. 303.520 and 303.521), if any, to parents of children eligible under this part.

(2) Consistent with Sec. 303.344(d), services provided pursuant to this section will include an educational component that promotes school readiness and incorporates preliteracy, language, and numeracy skills.

(3) The State policy will not affect the right of any child served pursuant to this section to receive FAPE (as that term is defined at Sec. 303.15) under Part B of the Act instead of early intervention services under Part C of the Act.

(4) Subject to Sec. 303.430(e), all early intervention services outlined in the child's IFSP under Sec. 303.344 will be continued while any eligibility determination is being made for services under this section.

(5) Informed consent must be obtained from the parents of any child to be served under this section, where practicable, before the child reaches three years of age, as to whether the parents intend to choose the continuation of early intervention services pursuant to this section for their child.

(6) The transition timeline requirements under Sec. 303.209(c)(1) and (d)(2) do not apply with respect to a child who is receiving services under this section until not fewer than 90 days—and, at the discretion of all of the parties, not more than nine months—before the time the child is expected to no longer receive services under this section.

(7) In States that adopt the option to make services under this part available to children ages three and older, there will be a referral to the Part C system dependent upon parental consent, of a child under the age of three who directly experiences a substantiated case of trauma due to exposure to family violence (as defined in Sec. 320 of the Family Violence Prevention and Services Act, 42 U.S.C. 10401 et seq.).

What activities can physical therapists specifically address for a child transitioning from early intervention?

Sample transition activities for a child with cerebral palsy who uses a power wheelchair for mobility and is transitioning to a community preschool program at age 3 years, could include, but not be limited to:

- providing information to the family to assure they understand community placement options so they can make informed decisions;
- initiating and participating in communication among the family and staff and related services personnel in the new environment(s) to understand daily routines, expectations of the adults and peers, and other demands in the future environment(s);
- providing onsite assessment and intervention to assure accessibility in the new environment and any other known environments the child frequently visits;
- providing assessment and intervention to assure that the child can be safely transported to desired environments by the family and preschool personnel;
- providing onsite assessment and identification of any new or different assistive technology needs of the child in the new environment(s);
- assisting in attaining any needed assistive technology;
- providing onsite consultation and training for the family and staff related to present and desired levels of functioning of the child in the new environment(s);
- providing onsite consultation and training for staff related to peers in the new environment(s);
- participating in the transition planning conference;
- participating in the transition IFSP/IEP meetings; and
- providing consultation following the transition to ensure that recommendations are useful and the child is successful.

In general, what is a physical therapist's role in transition for students throughout their school years?

Physical therapists may assume multiple roles throughout the transition process from Part C to Part B or in postsecondary transition. Regardless of the child's age, a primary goal is to ensure that the student is functioning in a meaningful way at the highest level of independence possible across relevant (inclusive) environments. Therefore, all IEP team members, including physical therapists, must individualize services based on the preferences, interests, skills, and unique needs of each student being served.[9] Ecological assessment of potential placement environment(s) is an important step along the way, including the anticipation and identification of any assistive technology needs, or consultation and training needs of significant adults and peers in those environments.[10]

Even though the definition of physical therapy in IDEA is broad—"services provided by a qualified physical therapist" (Sec. 300.34[c][9])—IDEA 2004 helps guide practices for children transitioning from early intervention into school-based programs and from high school to post-school activities.

What does transition from school to post-school activities involve?

Transition to post-school activities and adulthood can be described as "a dynamic, lifelong process that seeks to meet (students' with disabilities) individual needs as they move from childhood to adulthood."[11(p1304)] Transition is also a "process of gradual adoption of new roles and modification of existing roles" [12(p198)] for all students and their families. The underlying philosophy of IDEA 2004 reflects policymakers' desire for transition teams to consider supports that students with disabilities may need to benefit from transition services. In addition to providing supports to increase skills and promote transition goal attainment for youth with disabilities, physical therapy (as a related service) can enable access to integrated work, education, or adult living environments and experiences.[9]

The results-oriented transition focus of IDEA 2004 is strong in comparison to preceding legislation, and incorporates an educational shift in perspective from simply providing adult services to a transition perspective that promotes educational programs and curricular activities that are (1) based on students' post-high school goals and (2) driven by individual needs, interests, and preferences.[13-16] This perspective presumes that transition planning is a foundation from which to build educational programs and activities for students with disabilities, not just an add-on program for students when they reach age 16.

Kohler's *Taxonomy for Transition Programming*[17] provides a framework for students, families, teachers, and therapists to use in planning for and improving postsecondary outcomes for youth with disabilities. This taxonomy is based on literature reviews and research seeking to identify effective secondary transition practices.[17-20] The taxonomy's multilevel conceptual framework organizes effective transition practices according to the following 5 activity categories: (1) student-focused planning, (2) student development, (3) interagency collaboration, (4) family involvement, and (5) program structure.[17] Although related services may be provided within any level of the taxonomy, they are specifically implicated in the "student development" category. The expectation is that some students will require these services, including physical therapy, to achieve their postsecondary outcomes. The following section specifically details new legislative language that reflects the emphasis on postsecondary transition for youth with disabilities under Part B.

What is the new language on postsecondary transition?

Transition-focused activities may begin while a student is in middle or high school; however, IDEA specifically addresses activities and needs of students as they approach adulthood. According to Sec. 300.43, transition services means:

> *(a) … a coordinated set of activities for a child with a disability that—*
>
> *(1) Is designed within a results-oriented process, that is focused on improving the academic and functional achievement of the child with a disability to facilitate the child's movement from school to post-school activities, including postsecondary education, vocational education, integrated employment (including supported employment), continuing and adult education, adult services, independent living, or community participation;*
>
> *(2) Is based on individual child's needs, taking into account the child's strengths, preferences, and interests; and includes—*

(i) Instruction;
(ii) Related services;
(iii) Community experiences;
(iv) The development of employment and other post-school adult living objectives; and
(v) If appropriate, the acquisition of daily living skills and provision of a functional vocational evaluation.

(b) Transition services for children with disabilities may be special education, if provided as specially designed instruction, or a related service, if required to assist a child with a disability to benefit from special education.

Each state's State Performance Plan Indicators (#13, "Transition Components," and #14, "Transition Outcomes") help IEP teams determine if postsecondary goals are included and if they are accomplished after youth graduate from high school.[21]

What kind of postsecondary transition services are described on the IEP?

The transition IEP is a blueprint that helps students and their families, teachers, and other providers plan for postsecondary employment, education, and adult living.[22] According to Sec. 300.320(b):

> *Beginning not later than the first IEP to be in effect when the child turns 16, or younger if determined appropriate by the IEP Team, and updated annually, thereafter, the IEP must include—*
> *(1) appropriate measurable postsecondary goals based upon age appropriate transition assessments related to training, education, employment, and, where appropriate, independent living skills; and*
> *(2) the transition services needed to assist the child in reaching those goals.*

IDEA encourages planning for the changes that occur during postsecondary transition to simplify the transition planning process and to promote successful post-school career, education, and adult living opportunities for students with disabilities when they graduate.[23]

The convener of the initial transition meeting must indicate that the purpose of the meeting is to consider the student's postsecondary goals and transition services related to Sec. 300.320(b) (above). Furthermore, along with the rest of the IEP team, the school must invite the student and any other agency representative (or person) who might be instrumental in the youth's transition from high school.

Who is responsible when other agencies, such as the state vocational rehabilitation, are involved?

IDEA encourages interagency collaboration:

> *To the extent appropriate, with the consent of the parents or a child who has reached the age of majority, in implementing the requirements of paragraph (b)(1) of same section, the public agency must invite a representative of any participating agency that is likely to be responsible for providing or paying for transition services. (Sec. 300.321[b])*

The LEA is responsible, however, for ensuring the transition objectives are met. Sec. 300.324(c) says:

> *(1) If a participating agency, other than the public agency, fails to provide the transition services described in the IEP in accordance with Sec. 300.320(b), the public agency must reconvene the IEP Team to identify alternative strategies to meet the transition objectives for the child set out in the IEP.*
> *(2) Nothing in this part relieves any participating agency, including a State vocational rehabilitation agency, of the responsibility to provide or pay for any transition service that the agency would otherwise provide to children with disabilities who meet the eligibility criteria of that agency.*

Can transition services to post-school activities be provided for a student prior to the age of 16?

Yes. As the language above indicates, transition services are to begin no later than age 16 years, but may begin at a younger age if the IEP team determines that the student needs for transition services to begin sooner. Many states choose to begin transition services for younger students,[24] but are under no obligation to do so. Given that IEP team decisions must be individualized, the phrase "or younger if determined appropriate by the IEP Team" was included in Sec. 300.320(b).

What is a physical therapist's role in postsecondary transition?

Kohler's Taxonomy clearly implicates physical therapy as a support service that may be required as part of "student development" as youth pursue postsecondary transition visions.[13,14] Physical therapy services and supports for the student and for the IEP team can be provided through assessment, consultation, direct services, or any combination.[25] Physical therapists' roles in the transition process are to provide input on students' physical capacities, modifying daily activities, and/or designing, fabricating, or prescribing adaptive equipment to enable performance in the students' chosen community settings.[25] The Taxonomy gives many good examples of therapists' involvement in postsecondary transition activities such as identification and acquisition of assistive technology for postsecondary employment or education, assessment of a student's mobility relative to job requirements, and assisting students and their families with independent or supported adult living.[13,14] For students in high school, related environments should include postsecondary educational institutions, job sites, or adult living settings. Continued support across environments is essential to ensure the students' success in the new environment(s).[25]

Sec. 300.107 provides physical therapists with guidance for intervention in nonacademic settings at the time of students' transitions from high school. According to this section:

(a) *Each public agency must take steps, including the provision of supplementary aids and services determined appropriate and necessary by the child's IEP Team, to provide nonacademic and extracurricular services and activities in the manner necessary to afford children with disabilities an equal opportunity for participation in those services and activities.*

(b) *Nonacademic and extracurricular services and activities may include counseling services, athletics, transportation, health services, recreational activities, special interest groups or clubs sponsored by the public agency, referrals to agencies that provide assistance to individuals with disabilities, and employment of students, including both employment by the public agency and assistance in making outside employment available.*

What transition activities can physical therapists specifically address for students approaching the age of 16 or older?

An example of transition responsibilities for a physical therapist serving a 16-year-old student who has cerebral palsy and who plans to attend a local junior college and live independently in the community following graduation from high school might include, but not be limited to:

- initiating and participating in communication between the family and staff in the new environment(s) to understand daily routines, expectations of the adults and peers, and the demands of the future environment(s) (this communication should begin with the disabilities office at the community college);
- initiating contact and collaborating with the student's vocational rehabilitation counselor;
- providing onsite assessment and intervention to assure the student's ability to successfully maneuver around campus;
- providing assessment and intervention to access and use community transportation services;
- providing onsite consultation and training for the student, family, and appropriate staff related to present and desired levels of functioning for the student in the new environment(s) (eg, self-care skills, employment needs and options, grocery shopping, and accessing and participating in leisure activities);
- providing onsite assessment and identification of any new or different assistive technology needs of the student in the new environment(s);
- assisting in attaining any needed assistive technology;
- providing consultation and training for staff related to peer issues in the new environment(s) (eg, roommates and classmates);
- attending IEP meetings; and
- providing consultation following the transition to assure recommendations are effective and that the student is successful.

SUMMARY

Hains et al[1] described transition as a stressful time for children with disabilities and their families. Even with substantial preparation, many young children, students, and families are anxious about changing environments and service providers, and attending new programs. Physical therapists can help to make the transition from early intervention to school and from school to post-school activities as smooth and effective as possible. Understanding the needs of young children, students, and families in the new environments is essential for this transition. This means being present with students in their new environments, assessing and employing strategies for intervention in these environments, and consulting with staff and families regarding their concerns, suggestions, and expectations related to the new environments.

REFERENCES

1. Hains AH, Rosenkoetter SE, Fowler SA. Transition planning with families in early intervention programs. *Inf Young Child.* 1991;3(4):38-47.
2. Noonan MJ, Ratokalau NB. Project profile PPT: the preschool preparation and transition project. *J Early Intervent.* 1991;15(4):390-398.
3. Rosenkoetter SE, Hains AH, Fowler SA. *Bridging Early Services for Children with Special Needs and Their Families: A Practical Guide for Transition Planning.* Baltimore, MD: Paul H. Brookes; 1994.
4. Spiegel-McGill P, Reed DJ, Konig CS, McGowan PA. Parent education: easing the transition to preschool. *Top Early Child Spec Educ.* 1990;9(4):66-77.
5. Rous B, Hemmeter ML,Schuster J. Sequenced transition to education in the public schools: a systems approach to transition planning. *Top Early Child Spec Educ.* 1994;14(3):374-393.
6. Byrd MR, Rous BS. *Helpful Entry Level Skills Checklist–Revised.* Lexington, KY; Child Development Centers of the Bluegrass;1991.
7. Byrd MR, Rous BS. *Project STEPS: Instructional Manual for the Helpful Entry Level Skills Checklist.* 3rd ed. Lexington, KY; Child Development Centers of the Bluegrass;1997.
8. Noonan MJ, Ratokalau NB, Lauth-Torres L, McCormick L, Esaki CA, Claybaugh KW. Validating critical skills for preschool success. *The Transdisciplinary Journal.* 1992;2(3):187-203.
9. Simmons T, Flexor RW, Bauder D. (2005). Transition services. In: Flexer RW, Simmons TJ, Luft P, Baer RM, eds. *Transition Planning for Secondary Students With Disabilities.* Upper Saddle River, NJ: Pearson Education; 2005:203-229.
10. Inge K. *A National Survey of Occupational Therapists in the Public Schools: An Assessment of Current Practice, Attitudes, and Training Needs Regarding the Transition Process for Students With Severe Disabilities* [dissertation] Richmond, VA: Virginia Commonwealth University; 1995.
11. Blum R, Hirsch D, Kastner TA, Quint RD, Sandler AD. A consensus statement on health care transitions for young adults with special health care needs. *Pediatr.* 2002;110(6):1304-1306.
12. King GA, Baldwin PJ, Currie M, Evans J. Planning successful transitions from school to adult roles for youth with disabilities. *Children's Health Care.* 2005;34:193-216.
13. Clark GM, Kolstoe OP. *Career Development and Transition Education for Adolescents With Disabilities.* 2nd ed. Needham, MA: Allyn & Bacon; 1995.
14. Edgar E, Polloway EA. Education for adolescents with disabilities: curriculum and placement issues. *J Spec Educ.* 1994;27(4):438-452.
15. Gajar A, Goodman L, McAfee J. *Secondary Schools and Beyond: Transition of Individuals With Mild Disabilities.* Upper Saddle River, NJ: Merrill/Prentice Hall; 1993.
16. Rusch FR, DeStefano L, Chadsey-Rusch J, Phelps LA, Szymanski E. *Transition From High School to Adult Life: Models, Linkages, and Policy.* Sycamore, IL: Sycamore; 1992.
17. Kohler P. *A Taxonomy for Transition Programming: Linking Research and Practice.* Urbana-Champaign, IL: University of Illinois Transition Research Institute; 1996.
18. Kohler PD. Best practices in transition: substantiated or implied? *Career Dev Except Individuals.* 1996;16:107-121.
19. Kohler PD, DeStefano L, Wermuth TR, GraysonTE, McGinty S. An analysis of exemplary transition programs: how and why are they selected? *Career Dev Except Individuals.* 1994;17:187-202.
20. Rusch FR, Kohler PD, Hughes L. An analysis of OSERS-sponsored secondary special education and transitional services research. *Career Dev Except Individuals.* 1992;15:121-143.
21. National Secondary Transition Technical Assistance Center. Cross-referencing the Taxonomy for Transition Programming with NASET National Standards and Quality Indicators, 2007. http://www.nsttac.org/. Accessed July 11, 2007.

22. Sylvester L, Woods LL, Martin JE, Poolaw S. *Student-directed transition planning.* http://www.ok-ahead.org/test/index.html. Accessed April 4, 2007.

23. Stodden RA, Roberts KD. Transition legislation and policy: past and present. In: Rusch FR, ed. *Beyond High School: Preparing Adolescents for Tomorrow's Challenges.* 2nd ed. Upper Saddle River, NJ: Pearson Education; 2008:25-53.

24. Grack A. *What States Either Have, or Plan to Adopt, Legislative or Regulatory Language Requiring Secondary Transition.* Minneapolis, MN: North Central Regional Resource Center; 2005.

25. Shepherd J, Inge KJ. Occupational and physical therapy. In: deFur SH, Patton JR, eds. *Transition and School-based Services: Interdisciplinary Perspectives for Enhancing the Transition Process.* Austin, TX: PRO-ED; 1999:117-165.

8
Early Intervention Services in Natural Environments

Thubi H A Kolobe, PT, PhD, Lynn Jeffries, PT, PhD, PCS, and Julie D Smith, MS, OTR/L

One of the key provisions in Part C of IDEA is that early intervention must occur in children's natural environments. The overarching assumption is that providing interventions in the child's environment increases parent and child participation and promotes meaningful outcomes.[1]

What does "natural environment" mean?

According to Sec. 303.26:

> *Natural environments mean settings that are natural or normal for an infant or toddler without a disability, may include the home, and must be consistent with the provisions of Sec. 303.126.*

Sec. 303.126 says that early intervention services for infants and toddlers with disabilities must be provided:

> *(a) To the maximum extent appropriate, in natural environments; and*
>
> *(b) In settings other than the natural environment that are most appropriate, as determined by the parent and the IFSP team, only when early intervention services cannot be provided satisfactorily in a natural environment.*

Bruder and Dunst[2] have reframed the definition of natural environment to include the terms natural learning environments and natural learning opportunities. These authors conceptualized the terms as an approach to supporting a child's learning through family and community life activities. They defined natural learning environments as the everyday experiences, events, and places that serve as a child's sources of learning opportunities. The results of 2 national surveys conducted by the authors indicated that parents identified at least 22 kinds of natural learning environments that could be categorized as family life or community life:

> **Family life:** family routines, parenting routines, child routines, literacy activities, physical play, play activities, entertainment activities, family rituals, family celebrations, socialization activities, gardening activities.
>
> **Community life:** family activities, family outings, play activities, community events, outdoor activities, recreation activities, children's attractions, art/entertainment activities, church/religious groups, organizations/groups, sports activities/events.

Why is distinguishing between natural environment and natural learning opportunities important?

Natural environments are interpreted differently by various authors. Part C offers limited direction but seems to suggest that natural environments are related to a setting, such as the child's home or child care center. The APTA Section on Pediatrics[3] also describes a natural environment as a physical setting. Other authors, such as Hanft and Pilkington[4] and Dunst et al,[5] include the child's opportunities for learning as part of the definition of natural environments. A pattern that seems to have emerged from this literature (and not research) is that early writings described a natural environment as a setting. More recent literature tends to use an expanded version of the definition that includes natural learning opportunities. The differences in how the term is used may contribute to the inconsistent definitions of natural environments in the research literature, the difficulty in comparing studies, and differences in intervention approaches used. An important distinction is that adding natural learning opportunities to the conceptualization of natural environments shifts the focus more towards contextualized learning and less on the physical setting. This conceptualization moves early intervention providers to think beyond only the place in which services occur.

Natural learning opportunities occur within family and community life activities. For example, family routines offer learning opportunities through bedtime rituals such as choosing pajamas, bathing, putting on pajamas, brushing teeth, choosing a book for dad to read, and getting in bed. These activities can take place in a child's home, at a grandparent's home, or in other environments. Within each of these learning opportunities, however, a physical therapist can focus on different child skills based on the child's needs. For example during the bedtime ritual, depending on the child's needs and family goals, the father may help the child practice getting in and out of the bathtub, pulling pajamas out of a drawer, looking in the mirror and making facial expressions during teeth brushing, choosing a book by naming favorite characters, or pulling up bed covers in a playful manner. In this example the natural learning opportunities and the learning activities are varied but contextual, and occur in one natural setting.

Does the natural environment need to be included in the IFSP?

The team must document the setting of the early intervention services on the IFSP, as well as a justification of any services not provided in a natural environment. Sec. 303.344(d)(1)(ii) says the IFSP will include:

(A) *The natural environment setting in which early intervention services will be provided (subject to paragraph (d)(1)(ii)(B) of this section)*, *including, if applicable, a justification of the extent, if any, to which an early intervention service will not be provided in a natural environment.*

(B) *The determination of the appropriate setting for providing early intervention services to an infant or toddler with a disability, including any justification for not providing a particular early intervention service in the natural environment for that child and service, must be—*

(1) *Made by the IFSP team (which includes the parent and other team members);*

(2) *Consistent with the provisions in Sec. 303.13(a)(8), 303.26, and 303.126; and*

(3) *Based on the child's outcomes that are identified by the IFSP team in paragraph (c).*

Are community-based centers that provide interventions for children considered natural environments?

The question about whether centers that provide services for children with disabilities should be considered natural environments merits discussion. Centers that exclusively serve children with disabilities, even if based in the community, do not match the definition of natural environments. What is key in the discourse about natural environments should be whether or not children with and without disabilities have access to such settings, the context of the child's setting or activity, and the extent to which parents are involved in decision making. Community centers such as the YMCA, ballet class, or gymnastic schools could be considered natural environments if interventions are directed at the natural learning opportunities that ordinarily take place in these settings, and if the centers cater to all children. Although such center-based community programs may offer physical therapists opportunities to embed services in naturally occurring learning situations, an important distinction is that the learning activities that occur in these setting are not solely dependent on the physical therapist's presence.

What are the benefits of providing services in the natural environment?

Various authors have cited many benefits of providing interventions in natural environments,[4,6,7] some of which may also apply to other settings. The benefits that are unique to natural settings include: (1) increased opportunities to learn skills in a location and context where children will use them; (2) identification of barriers or constraints to skill acquisition; (3) the opportunity to observe family interactions; and (4) the opportunity to observe physical resources such as types of toys and space. Such opportunities maybe limited in center-based physical therapy programs. In the case of preschool children, providing services in the natural environments may have indirect benefits such as raising awareness about disability, empathy, and promoting friendships. Because the setting does not guarantee that the benefits will be realized, physical therapists need to be creative in how they maximize the use of these environments. For example, while putting on pajamas is a naturally occurring event among children, teaching a child this skill in the middle of the day may be out of context. In this case the physical therapist may need to decide first whether barriers associated with task are unique to putting on pajamas. In many cases other natural learning opportunities, such as changing clothes for swimming, are likely to present difficulties similar to putting on pajamas.

What are the limitations and disadvantages of providing services in natural environments?

Most of the disadvantages have to do with provider support, safety, and productivity; institutional financial constraints; and parents' access to parent support groups. Provider support may be limited because opportunities for collaboration and communication among providers, although not guaranteed in other settings such as center-based programs, are limited. Physical therapists need to make more effort to communicate and collaborate than if they were working in the same physical setting. Another disadvantage that often is mentioned is risky households and neighborhoods with high crime. Although the solutions are not easy, the consensus appears to be for programs to emphasize training for personal safety, preplanning visits, and scheduling early morning appointments, and on the extreme end, using escorts and buddy systems.[8,9] Some of the recommended strategies, however, may compromise family-professional collaboration.

Parent support may be more limited when services are provided in natural environment because, unlike center-based programs that routinely offer a variety of parent groups that are easily accessible to parents, many of the programs that provide interventions in natural environments rely on informal parent-to-parent groups. Depending on when and where the groups are scheduled, parents may have problems using them routinely for support.

Another disadvantage relates to providers' working schedules. For example, family routines or natural learning opportunities in which children participate occur over the course of the day and evening. The timing may make it difficult for professionals to schedule extended times not only to observe the events, but also to identify and recommend practice opportunities that are likely to promote functional skills. Many physical therapists use set weekly schedules (eg, 1 or 2 times per week), which provide a limited window for gathering information about what happens in a child's life during the week. It is important that physical therapists recognize these limitations and, when indicated, seek ways to use or advocate for flexible scheduling.

The disadvantage of services in natural environments for children pertains to the use of specialized equipment for intervention, if required, and the possibility for peer interactions during group interventions. Toddler group interventions are logistically difficult to infuse in programs that provide intervention only in the child's home, which challenges physical therapists to be creative about ways to maximize peer interactions while providing intervention in natural environments.

How should assessment and interventions be provided in the natural environment?

Part C defines assessment of service needs as the planning process used to identify the child's and family's needs (Sec. 303.320[d]). The identified needs become the basis for the IFSP outcomes and intervention strategies discussed in Chapter 5. The details about how assessments should be conducted in natural environment are left up to service providers. How and what the child is doing or has difficulties doing within their natural learning environments should form a central part of assessment, and may indeed be the single most defining factor that differentiates between the findings obtained from assessment of naturally occurring activities within the natural environments and from non-inclusive center-based settings. Assessment should include, but not limited to, the following 4 steps:

1. Interview the family or caregivers for the purpose of information exchange and for the therapist to learn about how the family has helped the child participate in the naturally occurring learning opportunities in family and community routines and activities. To capture the richness of how the caregiving environment creates and could use natural learning opportunities, therapists need to expand their listening skills beyond words to meaning.
2. Observe and discuss how the child participates in the naturally occurring family or community routines and within natural environments (eg, eating breakfast, expressing needs and wants, playing with other children or with caregivers, bathing, and dressing) to determine barriers. Barriers to participation may be related to limitations in the child's activities or impairments in body structure and functions.10 To identify limitations in activities or body structures and functions, physical therapists should use reliable and valid standardized tests and measures supplemented by clinical observations.
3. Introduce intervention strategies and activities to the learning opportunities for the purpose of testing whether they can enhance the child's participation. This involves incorporating and building upon ideas, strategies, and activities that the family and other care providers have used. An example is a family that likes to spend time outside and would like the child to play on a swing with his brother. The child may have difficulty holding on to the swing or holding her head up when the swing is in motion. During the assessment, the physical therapist could first adapt the environment by trying different seating inserts with head supports and observing if the child can hold on to the swing. Depending on the outcome, the physical therapist may add supports for the arms and hands. If the performance does not change, the physical therapist would then focus on person factors such as muscle weakness and potential for improvement if alleviated.
4. Establish a common understanding among caregivers and professionals of what the child can and cannot do, and why, natural learning opportunities that can be targeted for intervention, and intended or expected outcomes. This step entails interpreting the findings or information from the interviews, observations, tests and measures; speculating or hypothesizing on factors that contribute to limitations in participation or activity; and analyzing decisions.

These 4 steps are also a part of the IFSP process and document.

How should interventions be provided in the natural environment?

Intervention is a collaborative effort that seeks to use as many natural learning opportunities as feasible. Priority should be given to interventions that resulted from the common understanding of expectations and outcomes. Because intervention is based on continuous assessment, each visit or intervention session should involve exchange of ideas and suggestions between the caregivers and physical therapists. During intervention, assessment focuses on the caregiver's appraisal of which intervention strategies have worked or have not worked. Decisions about whether to continue implementing the same strategies, modify all or part of the strategies, or expand the strategies for new learning opportunities are based on a team decision. The team includes the family, other caregivers, and service providers involved in the implementation of the IFSP. The focus is on helping parents and other caregivers maximize their confidence and abilities so child learning and development of new skills occurs naturally as a part of everyday life.[2,11,12]

Literature describes several approaches and strategies that are intended to maximize information gathering and exchange as part of assessment and intervention.[7,13,14] An in-depth discussion of these approaches is beyond the scope of this chapter. Examples are teaching and learning strategies such as coaching and participatory guidance. Coaching is an interaction style between therapists and the family that allows the therapist to help the family build competence and confidence[12] and simultaneously allows the therapist to gain information from the family. The components of coaching include: joint planning, observation, action/practice, reflection, and feedback. For more information on these components please see Rush and Shelden[15] and Rush et al.[12]

The concept of guided participation comes from Vytskofsy's theory of social learning,[16] which Rogoff later revived.[17] Participatory guidance, as a form of learning and teaching, centers on information exchange as a shared endeavor that is organized around a specific area or activity, making the process a joint enterprise between learner and teacher.[17] It is intended to provide a way to look at how 2 people engage in a process of attaining a common understanding of an activity or task,[14] help bridge the known to the new,[17] and understand meaning from another's perspective.[18] Participatory guidance is similar to what parents do when they teach their children culturally valued practices or activities. For example, parents structure and guide the child's learning experiences in novel and routine situations by adjusting the level of the child's participation based on the child's increasing skill.

What are some examples?

Using this instructional approach, and to ensure mutual understanding and structuring, a physical therapist would first have to learn how's and why's of the teaching styles (from the child's parents or caregiver), seek for meaning before offering suggestions about targeted learning situations or goals, and offer suggestions that focus on expanding the parents' current understanding to a new level. An example would be an 18-month-old child with spastic quadriplegic cerebral palsy, whose goals on the IFSP include "increased use of hands." During discussions with the caregiver, the physical therapist may learn that one of the child's favorite rituals is bed-time or nap-time reading (natural learning opportunity). Instead of offering suggestions for how to increase the child's use of arms, such as pointing at pictures, the physical therapist would engage the parent in the discussion about this ritual, the expected role for the child, and significance of verbal and nonverbal communication to the family. The physical therapist can use the responses as references upon which to expand. If the parents' teaching repertoire involves putting a child on their laps and turning the pages of the book while the child quietly listens, suggestions can center around various ways to encourage the child to turn pages. In essence, participatory guidance may promote the physical therapist's full understanding of the caregiving environment and meaning, and using this knowledge as leverage for the development of new and shared ideas.

Other examples of natural learning opportunities that occur in the natural environment and that could be considered shared endeavors are bathing and dressing, meals, putting children to bed, or play. Although activities such as these are quite common practices, how they are performed with children with disabilities may be unique for each family and professional, and may require a great deal of caregiver–professional information exchange. For example, the caregiver and professional may differ in their understanding of how to carry out these activities with children who are medically fragile and developmentally vulnerable.

Physical therapists providing services under Part C must remember that the focus is to bridge the understanding between themselves and families and to provide assessments and interventions that enhance this understanding. Partnering with, and supporting a family's influence on their child's development is key to providing services in natural environments under IDEA. As discussed previously, this also requires making explicit the distinction between natural environments and naturally occurring learning opportunities or routines. If the natural environment is the place where the child and family routines take place, and naturally occurring activities are the routines, then providing intervention in natural environment should capitalize on naturally occurring events in the natural environment (contextual).

Providing intervention in the natural environments still requires physical therapists to engage in sound, evidence-based decision making.[19] Providers who use evidence to support recommended activities and seek creative ways to enrich the learning environment are more likely to be effective regardless of the physical context in which intervention is provided.

What is the evidence that supports providing intervention in the natural environment?

Much of the current literature on natural environments fosters an understanding of why providing services in natural environments is important and offers suggestions for implementation.[4,6,20,21] This literature relies heavily on secondary sources. Initially the research that shaped the arguments for natural environments came from research findings in psychology about role of consistency and repetitions in fostering learning and mastery,[5] programs that showed transitionary increase in IQ scores among children considered to be at risk for developmental delays or disabilities,[22] and findings described in the Neurons to Neighborhood Report.[23] These research studies used a variety of models and approaches that differed in terms of operational definitions, characteristics, and assumptions about natural environments. The focus of much of the research was on identifying and understanding the characteristics of environments that influenced child outcome. Therefore, current recommendations for intervention are based largely on extrapolations of a combination of these findings rather than studies that have directly tested models of natural environment intervention to determine their efficacy.

Following a review of 166 articles, many of which have been used to support intervention models in natural environments, Dunst et al[5] concluded:

> *Unfortunately we do not know exactly, or even imprecisely, what constitutes a logical mix of natural learning environments practices because research has not been conducted on the makeup of the combinations of practices at different child ages and under different conditions. This type of research is sorely needed.*(p57).

Regarding the need to use a variety of contextually based learning opportunities rather than providing services in one setting, the authors wrote[5]:

> *States' movement toward institutionalization of this narrow interpretation of natural environments needs to be redirected if the best interests of the children and families are to be served by natural learning environment practices. This is especially true in light of the fact that research on this kind of practice is essentially nonexistent.*(p57)

What are the implications of lacking evidence for practice?

The paucity of research to support the effectiveness and efficacy of providing intervention in natural environments and targeting naturally occurring activities has implications for practice. First, it suggests that physical therapists cannot assume that providing therapy in natural environments implies that such interventions are effective. If anything, the limited findings underscore the need for physical therapists to continue seek ways not only to use a variety of teaching and learning strategies, but also to document the outcomes of such interventions in a manner that permits comparisons over time and across families. Second, physical therapists need to develop conceptual models that can be used to study the effectiveness of their role when services target natural learning opportunities in natural environments. Such models must be tested empirically.

Although the focus of this chapter is on providing physical therapy in natural environments, physical therapists need to be aware of the findings that compare home- vs. center-based interventions. Studies in this area that have often been cited in the past have shown mixed findings; however, a recent analysis[24] of large studies that have been conducted over the last decade with infants and toddlers with and without disabilities showed favorable developmental outcomes for programs that combined home- with center-based programs, compared to home-based or center-based programs alone. Often the home-based program focused on individualized activities and parent education during the first 2 years of life, whereas center-based programs, often initiated after 24 months, focused on structured and curriculum-based activities. This finding suggests the need for physical therapists to move beyond the philosophical to research-based intervention approaches and strategies. The natural environment includes context and multiple variables that contribute to the success of any intervention. The variables include the role of consistency and repetitions in fostering learning and mastery. It is not only the challenges that children encounter in natural environments that affect outcome, but also the frequency with which such encounters occur. The consistency and frequency may help explain the beneficial effects of natural environments that include center-based programs. Many typically developing children use both.

SUMMARY

Part C of IDEA says that early intervention must occur in children's natural environments. In this chapter we used the broad definition of natural environments proposed by Bruder and Dunst[2] and Dunst and colleagues[5] that includes natural learning opportunities. Physical therapists working in early intervention programs must consider the contextualized activities children participate in and not just the location of services. A physical therapist's ability to implement evidence-based and family-centered care is paramount regardless of the environment in which the care is provided.

REFERENCES

1. Bernheimer LP, Gallimore R, Weisner TS. Ecocultural theory as a context for the individual family service plan. *J Early Intervent.* 1990;14:219-233.
2. Bruder MB, Dunst CJ. Expanding learning opportunities for infants and toddlers in natural environments: a chance to reconceptualize early intervention. *Zero to Three.* 2000;20:34-36.
3. American Physical Therapy Association Section on Pediatrics Web site. Early intervention services: natural learning environments. http://www.pediatricapta.org/graphics/EIFactsheet.pdf. Accessed August 3, 2007.
4. Hanft B, Pilkington K. Therapy in natural environments: the means or end goal for early intervention? *Inf Young Child.* 2000;12(4):1-13.
5. Dunst CJ, Trivette CM, Humphries T, Raab M, Roper N. Contrasting approaches to natural learning environment interventions. *Inf Young Child.* 2001;14(2):48-63.
6. Shelden ML, Rush DD. The ten myths about providing early intervention services in natural environments. *Inf Young Child.* 2001;14(1):1-13.
7. Dunst CJ, Hamby D, Trivette CM, Raab M, Bruder M. Everyday family and community life and children's naturally occurring learning opportunities. *J Early Intervent.* 2000;23(3):151-164.
8. Kendra MA, Weiker A, Simon S, Grant A, Shullick D. Safety concerns affecting delivery of home health care. *Pub Health Nurs.* 1996;13(2):83-89.
9. Coke T, Alday R, Biala K, Luna S, Martines P. The new role of physical therapy in home care. *Home Healthcare Nurse: The Journal for the Home Care and Hospice Professional.* 2005;23(9):594-599.
10. World Health Organization. *International Classification of Functioning, Disability and Health: ICF.* Geneva, Switzerland: World Health Organization; 2001.
11. Hanft BE, Rush DD, Shelden ML. *Coaching Families and Colleagues in Early Childhood.* Baltimore, MD: Paul H. Brookes; 2004.
12. Rush DD, Shelden ML, Hanft B. Coaching families and colleagues: a process for collaboration in natural settings. *Inf Young Child.* 2003;15(3):27-41.
13. Kolobe THA, Taylor A. The environment of intervention. In: Campbell SK, VanderLinden DW, Palisano RJ, eds. *Physical Therapy for Children.* 3rd ed. Philadelphia, PA: Elsevier; 2006:909–932.
14. Rogoff B, Mistry J, Göncü A, Mosier C. Guided participation in cultural activity by toddlers and caregivers. *Monogr Soc Res Child Dev.* 1993;58(8):v-vi, 1-174; discussion 175-179.
15. Rush DD, Shelden ML. Evidenced-based definition of coaching practices. *CASEinPoint* [serial online]. 2005;1(6):1-6. http://www.fippcase.org/caseinpoint/ caseinpoint_vol1_no6.pdf. Accessed August 3, 2007.
16. Vytskofsky LS. *Mind in Society: The Development of Higher Psychological Processes.* Cambridge, MA. Harvard University Press; 1978.
17. Rogoff B. *Apprenticeship in Thinking: Cognitive Development in a Social Context.* New York, NY: Oxford University Press; 1990.
18. Rogoff B, Paradise R, Arauz RM, Correa-Chavez M, Angelillo C. Firsthand learning through intent participation. *Annu Rev Psychol.* 2003;54:175-203.
19. Palisano RJ, Campbell SK, Harris SR. Evidence-based decision making in pediatric physical therapy. In: Campbell SK, VanderLinden DW, Palisano RJ, eds. *Physical Therapy for Children.* 3rd ed. Philadelphia, PA: Elsevier; 2006:3-32.
20. Mu K, Royeen C. Facilitating participation of students with severe disabilities: aligning school-based occupational therapy with the best practice in severe disabilities. *Phys Occup Ther Pediatr.* 2004;24(3):5-21.
21. Wilson LL, Mott DW, Batman D. The asset-based context matrix: a tool for assessing children's learning opportunities and participation in natural environments. *Top Early Child Educ.* 2004;24(2):110-120.
22. Ramey CT, Bryant DM, Wasik BH, Sparling JJ, Fendt KH, La Vange LM. Infant Health and Development Program for low birth weight, premature infants: program elements, family participation, and child intelligence. *Pediatr.* 1992;89:454-465.
23. Shonkoff JP, Phillips DA, eds. For the Committee on Integrating the Science of Early Childhood Development, Board on Children, Youth, and Families. *From Neurons to Neighborhoods: The Science of Early Childhood Development.* Washington, DC: National Academies Press; 2000.
24. Gray R, McCormick MC. Early childhood intervention programs in the US: recent advances and future recommendations. *J Primary Prev.* 2005;26(3):259-275.

9 Intervention in the Schools

Irene McEwen, PT, PhD, FAPTA

How should physical therapists provide services in the schools?

Physical therapy is defined in IDEA as "services provided by a qualified physical therapist" (Sec. 300.34[c][9]). This definition supports any service within the physical therapist's scope of practice that the IEP team agrees is needed to "assist a child with a disability to benefit from special education" (Sec. 300.34[a]).

The *Guide to Physical Therapist Practice*[1] also provides guidance about intervention that is consistent with IDEA. The Guide defines intervention as:

> *... the purposeful interaction of the physical therapist with the patient/client, and when appropriate other individuals involved in the patient/client care, using various physical therapy procedures and techniques to produce changes in a condition that are consistent with the diagnosis and prognosis. Decisions about interventions are contingent on the timely monitoring of the patient/client response and progress make toward achieving anticipated goals and expected outcomes.*[(p38)]

The Guide describes 3 components of intervention, all of which are appropriate and important to consider in school-based practice: (1) coordination, communication, and documentation; (2) child-related instruction; and (3) procedural interventions.

What do coordination, communication, and documentation involve?

When working in schools, physical therapists never work in isolation; they are always members of children's education teams. Sometimes they are members of more than 1 team of a child, such as an education team and a medical team, and a physical therapist may serve as a liaison between the 2 teams. With parents, teachers, other related services providers, and other school personnel all involved with each child, coordination and communication among and between team members clearly is an essential part of providing school-based services.[2] Without good coordination of services and communication among team members, interventions are likely to overlap, have gaps, or even conflict—all of which could unnecessarily limit a child's achievement.

Documentation of school-based physical therapy services needs to follow local education agency (LEA) requirements, which reflect federal and state regulations and comply with the state's physical therapy practice act.[2] A LEA that seeks reimbursement from Medicaid or other payer may have additional requirements for documentation, which should apply to all children, not only those for whom reimbursement is sought.

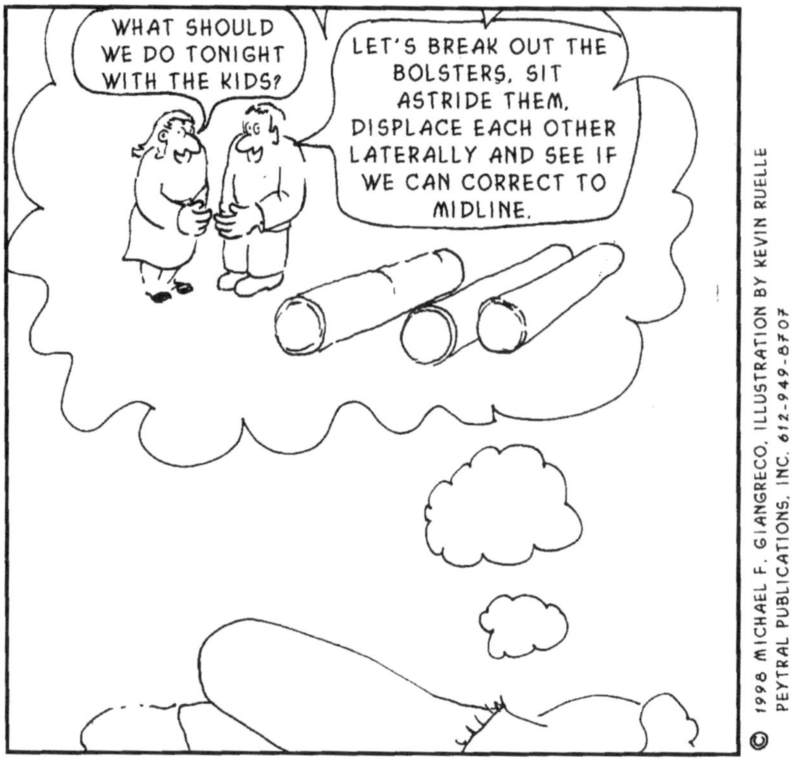
WHAT SHOULD WE DO TONIGHT WITH THE KIDS?
LET'S BREAK OUT THE BOLSTERS, SIT ASTRIDE THEM, DISPLACE EACH OTHER LATERALLY AND SEE IF WE CAN CORRECT TO MIDLINE.
© 1998 MICHAEL F. GIANGRECO, ILLUSTRATION BY KEVIN RUELLE
PEYTRAL PUBLICATIONS, INC. 612-949-8707

ONLY IN A PHYSICAL THERAPIST'S DREAM.

What does child-related instruction include?

The Guide defines "patient/client-related" instruction as "the process of informing, educating, or training patients/clients, families, significant others, and caregivers…to promote and optimize physical therapy services."[1(p39)] The Guide's definition is somewhat hierarchical, with the physical therapist doing the informing, educating, and training. In schools, a more collaborative process is necessary, with exchange of information among physical therapists and other team members important to identify and provide effective intervention. This process frequently is called collaborative consultation, and *The Consulting Therapist: A Guide for OTs and PTs in Schools*[3] is a helpful resource.

What procedural interventions are appropriate in schools?

Procedural interventions are specific procedures and techniques that physical therapists identify and provide for the child or, when appropriate, collaborate with other team members to provide. Examples of procedural interventions are therapeutic exercise, functional training, and assistive technology.[1] Any procedural interventions that are most likely to help a child achieve the goals and are within the scope of physical therapist practice would be appropriate. Team members should be aware, however, of a new requirement in IDEA 2004 that the IEP must include:

> *A statement of the special education and related services, supplementary aids and services, based on peer-reviewed research to the extent practicable, to be provided to the child. Sec. 300.320(a)(4)*

Regular monitoring of progress is important, with changes made if intervention is not helping the child achieve the goals within the projected timelines.

What does "peer-reviewed research to the extent practicable" mean?

The "Analysis of Comments and Changes" section of the *Federal Register* prior to the regulations (see the CD) helps to explain these terms:

"Peer-reviewed research" generally refers to research that is reviewed by qualified and independent reviewers to ensure that the quality of the information meets the standards of the field before the research is published. However, there is no single definition of "peer reviewed research" because the review process varies depending on the type of information to be reviewed.[71 FR 46664]
The phrase "to the extent practicable," as used in this context, generally means that services and supports should be based on peer-reviewed research to the extent that it is possible, given the availability of peer-reviewed research.[71 FR 46665]

Does this mean that the IEP team has to discuss peer-reviewed research before making decisions?

Although knowledge and discussion of relevant research obviously is important, the law does not require a "focused discussion"[71 FR 46665] about research or documentation of any discussion. The "Analysis of Comments and Changes" section of the regulations again is helpful:

> *We decline to require all IEP Team meetings to include a focused discussion on research-based methods or require public agencies to provide prior written notice when an IEP Team refuses to provide documentation of research-based methods, as we believe such requirements are unnecessary and would be overly burdensome.*[71 FR 46665]

How do requirements for peer-reviewed research to the extent practicable relate to FAPE?

The "Analysis and Comments" section of the regulations also addressed this question:

> *States, school districts, and school personnel must ...select and use methods that research has shown to be effective, to the extent that methods based on peer-reviewed research are available. This does not mean that the service with the greatest body of research is the service necessarily required for a child to receive FAPE. Likewise, there is nothing in the Act to suggest that the failure of public agency to provide services based on peer-reviewed research would automatically result in a denial of FAPE. The final decision about the special education and related services, and supplementary aids and services that are to be provided to a child must be made by the child's IEP Team based on the child's individual needs.* [71 FR 46665]

How does the requirement for peer-reviewed research to the extent practicable relate to evidence-based practice?

Evidence-based practice has become increasingly important in all areas of physical therapist practice. A common definition of evidence-based practice is the "integration of best research evidence with our clinical expertise and our patient's unique values and circumstances."[4] The best available research evidence usually is peer-reviewed, so that part of the definition is consistent with IDEA. The clinical expertise and patient's unique values and circumstance part of the definition is consistent with the authority that IDEA gives to the child's IEP team to make decisions based on the child's unique needs.

Does peer-reviewed research apply only to interventions?

No, physical therapists need to consider peer-reviewed research in each part of the physical therapist patient/client management process: examination, evaluation, diagnosis, prognosis, intervention, and outcomes measurement.[1] Each of the other components do, of course, influence decisions about intervention.

What is an example?

During the examination, a physical therapist might measure the joint range of motion of a child with cerebral palsy. Research is available on the reliability of goniometric measurements in children with cerebral palsy,[5-7] which would help estimate the amount of error that is likely in a measurement and the amount of change that could be considered real change. This information would then be used in the evaluation part of the process, when the physical therapist combines all examination information to make clinical judgments. A question to answer, for example, is has the child's range of motion decreased over time or are any measured differences likely to be due to measurement error? If they are likely to be due to measurement error, then decisions probably would be different than if changes are likely to be real.

Research on prognosis is important for predicting whether a child is likely to be able to achieve certain goals. Research is available, for example, to help predict ambulation[8] and gross motor development in children with cerebral palsy[9] and Down syndrome.[10] Although individual children can have personal and/or environmental characteristics that make their prognosis different than the grouped data in research reports, the results of studies on prognosis are important to know about, understand, and incorporate into decision making and discussions with other team members. A child with cerebral palsy classified at Level IV on the Gross Motor Function Classification System,[11] for example, is unlikely to walk without a great deal of support and will need assistance with mobility. Power mobility often is the best option. Research supports the stability of the children's classifications over time.[12]

Does much peer-reviewed research exist on procedural interventions?

A rapidly increasing body of research is available on procedural interventions that physical therapists commonly use. Although most of it is peer-reviewed, many of the studies are limited by small sample sizes and modest quality, at best. One of the most useful ways to learn about the effectiveness of interventions is to look for systematic reviews or meta-analyses, which combine results from several studies into one overall conclusion. Unfortunately, many systematic reviewers conclude that findings are inconclusive and we need more research, but the studies do provide more direction than no research at all. Systematic reviews are available on a number of procedural interventions, including: adapted seating for children with cerebral palsy[13,14]; conductive education[15]; constraint-induced movement therapy[16]; lower-extremity casting, orthoses, and splints for children with neurological disorders[17-20]; neurodevelopmental treatment[21-23]; partial body-weight–supported treadmill training[24]; passive stretching to improve range of motion[25,26]; strengthening for children with cerebral palsy[27,28]; and weight-bearing interventions for children with cerebral palsy.[29]

Do procedural interventions need to be one-to-one?

No, intervention may be provided for groups of students. A survey of pediatric physical therapists indicated that over 60% of respondents working in the schools used group intervention, particularly with young children with developmental delays.[30] The most common emphasis in these groups was task-specific activities, followed by developmental activities. The reported major benefit of group intervention was peer modeling.

What is integrated therapy?

Integrated therapy is based on a team-oriented approach to service delivery that promotes students' achievement of functional skills.[31] The entire team, including the family, participates in developing the student's goals and implementing intervention to achieve them. Rainforth and York-Barr[31] identified the following essential components for team members to consider when collaborating in the development and implementation of an integrated educational program:

1. *All goals and objectives belong to the learner, rather than to individual team members.*
2. *All team members are responsible for contributing information and skills that will maximize learner success in accomplishing all goals and objectives.*
3. *Each team member has specialized disciplinary methods and skills, many of which can be taught to other team members.*
4. *Combining methods from a variety of disciplines allows all team members to address the needs of the learner more successfully and in more natural contexts.*
5. *Individually selected, meaningful activities are the logical and necessary focus around which team members identify and integrate effective instructional methods for each learner.*[(p191)]

What are some examples of integrated therapy activities?

Integrated therapy activities are as varied as the creativity and commitment of the team. A physical therapist might, for example: (1) develop a seating system for a student in third grade so that the student can use the

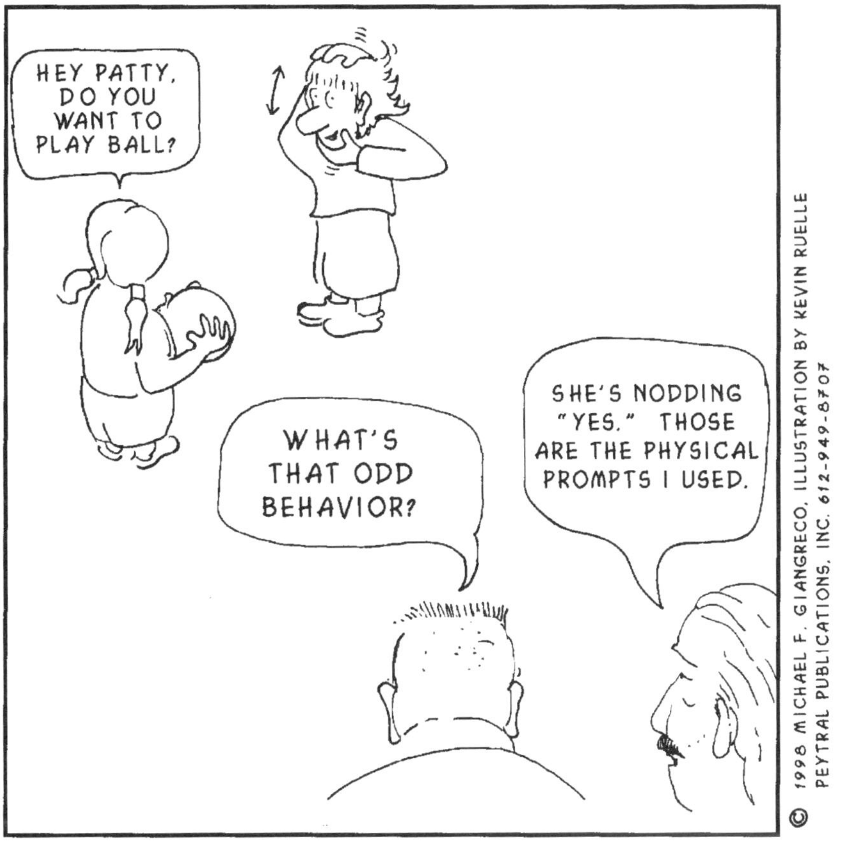
HEY PATTY, DO YOU WANT TO PLAY BALL?
WHAT'S THAT ODD BEHAVIOR?
SHE'S NODDING "YES." THOSE ARE THE PHYSICAL PROMPTS I USED.
© 1998 MICHAEL F. GIANGRECO, ILLUSTRATION BY KEVIN RUELLE
PEYTRAL PUBLICATIONS, INC. 612-949-8707

PATTY'S TEACHER RETURNED THE BOOK ON APPLIED BEHAVIOR ANALYSIS BEFORE HE HAD A CHANCE TO READ THE CHAPTER ON FADING PHYSICAL PROMPTS.

classroom computer, (2) assist a child in preschool to transfer out of his wheelchair to the carpet for story time, (3) help a student with visual and motor impairments to become independently mobile on a school campus, (4) teach a student with a traumatic brain injury to use the bathroom at school, or (5) support a student and his high school IEP team in the student's transition from school to work. Obviously, these activities would not be practiced in an isolated physical therapy room, but rather would be performed in the environments in which they naturally occur, such as the classroom, bathroom, school campus, or a job site.

When working in an integrated model, rarely does a physical therapist work only with a student; the PT also works with parents, teachers, paraprofessionals, and other team members who can provide students with multiple opportunities to practice motor skills in as many environments as the skill is needed. In this way, student have the opportunity to practice motor skills throughout each day, not only during therapy time.[32] The importance of intense practice was repeatedly emphasized during the III STEP Conference, sponsored by the American Physical Therapy Association's Neurology Section and Section on Pediatrics in 2005,[33,34] which focused on linking movement science and intervention. To provide opportunities for the amount of practice likely to improve children's skills, physical therapists must communicate and coordinate with other team members so others also can help students practice motor tasks.

Is it legal and ethical for others to provide physical therapy?

The other team members whom a physical therapist teaches do not provide physical therapy services. Rather, they carry out educational activities that the physical therapist recommends to help a child learn motor skills, function more effectively in the classroom, and so forth. This should not become a concern when goals are discipline-free and reflect a student's overall educational program. Classroom assistants, for example, do not work on "physical therapy goals."

Nothing in the American Physical Therapy Association (APTA) Code of Ethics[35] suggests teaching others is unethical and the *Guide to Physical Therapist Practice*[1] identifies "patient/client-related instruction" for families and other caregivers as a part of intervention. Although physical therapists must be familiar with their respective state practice acts, Rainforth[36] reviewed 51 practice acts and found nothing that would prevent physical therapists who work in school settings from delegating the kinds of tasks and methods provided as a related service. She concluded:

> *Documents that define the legal and ethical practice of physical therapy allow for, and even encourage role release in educational settings. The roles of evaluation, treatment planning, and supervision may not be delegated, but intervention may be carried out by others who are trained and supervised by a physical therapist. Although physical therapists must still determine what constitutes adequate training and supervision, therapists who resist role release due to concerns for their liability must also consider the potential risks to children and staff when therapeutic intervention is limited to isolated treatment sessions.*[36(p57)]

Obviously, physical therapists must use good judgment when deciding what to delegate and to whom to delegate and must provide appropriate training and monitoring. These procedures, like any other services, need to be thoroughly documented.

Where should physical therapy take place?

Physical therapy services rarely should be provided in a physical therapy room or other isolated setting. By definition, school-based physical therapy services assist a child with a disability to benefit from special education; therefore, physical therapists primarily should work in the classroom or other places in the school and/or community that support the student's special education program. Communication among the student's teachers and physical therapist is essential if the IEP goals and objectives are to be met, and communication is best accomplished when physical therapists and teachers work with students in the same locations.

Although conclusive evidence is not yet available to support the effectiveness of working with disabilities in classrooms and other natural environments, it is current best practice in pediatric physical therapy[37] and is supported by motor learning principles.[38] Much variability exists nationwide, however, with physical therapists in some parts of the country providing more isolated services for students in schools than physical therapists in other parts of the country.[39]

Do interventions need to be written on the IEP?

The IEP team may discuss specific interventions, but interventions are not documented on the IEP and may change when necessary without needing to revise the IEP. The exception is assistive technology, which does need to be documented.

SUMMARY

School-based physical therapy intervention for students with disabilities combines the requirements of IDEA, including peer-reviewed research, with evidence-base practice, the current best practices in pediatric physical therapy. School-based physical therapists need to be familiar with, understand, and apply research on examination, prognosis, and intervention to intervention decisions for students with disabilities. IDEA supports the use of motor learning principles, which suggest that intervention will be more effective if it takes place in the environments in which students need to use skills being taught and if physical therapists help parents, teachers, and other team members learn to promote students' motor skills during their daily interactions with them.

REFERENCES

1. *Guide to Physical Therapist Practice.* Revised 2nd ed. Alexandria, VA: American Physical Therapy Association; 2003.
2. Effgen SK. Schools. In: Effgen SK, ed. *Meeting the Physical Therapy Needs of Children.* Philadelphia, PA: FA Davis; 2005:361-376.
3. Hanft BE, Place PA. *The Consulting Therapist: A Guide for OTs and PTs in Schools.* San Antonio, TX: Harcourt Assessment; 1998.
4. Straus SE, Richardson WS, Glasziou P, Haynes RB. *Evidence-based Medicine: How to Practice and Teach EBM.* 3rd ed. New York, NY: Churchill Livingstone; 2005.
5. Kilgour G, McNair P, Stott NS. Intrarater reliability of lower limb sagittal range-of-motion measures in children with spastic diplegia. *Dev Med Child Neurol.* 2003;45:391-399.
6. McWhirk LB. Glanzman AM. Within-session inter-rater reliability of goniometric measures in patients with spastic cerebral palsy. *Pediatr Phys Ther. 2006;18:262-265.*
7. Stuberg WA, Fuchs RH, Miedaner JA. Reliability of goniometric measurements of children with cerebral palsy. *Dev Med Child Neurol. 1988;30:657-666.*
8. Campos du Paz A, Burnett S, Braga, L. Walking prognosis in cerebral palsy. *Dev Med Child Neur*ol. 1994;36:130-134.
9. Rosenbaum PL, Walter SD, Hanna SE, et al. Prognosis for gross motor function in cerebral palsy: creation of motor development curves. *JAMA.* 2002;288:1357-1363.
10. Palisano RJ, Walter SD, Russell DJ, et al. Gross motor function of children with Down syndrome: creation of motor growth curves. *Arch Phys Med Rehabil.* 2001;82:494-500.
11. Palisano R, Rosenbaum P, Walter S, Russell D, Wood E, Galuppi B. Gross Motor Function Classification System. *Dev Med Child Neurol.* 1997;39:214-223.
12. Palisano RJ, Cameron D, Rosenbaum PL, Walter SD, Russell D. Stability of the Gross Motor Function Classification System. *Dev Med Child Neurol. 2006;48:424-428.*
13. Harris SR, Roxborough L. Efficacy and effectiveness of physical therapy in enhancing postural control in children with cerebral palsy. *Neural Plasticity.* 2005;12(2-3):229-243.
14. Roxborough L. Review of the efficacy and effectiveness of adaptive seating for children with cerebral palsy. *Assistive Technology.* 1995;*7:17-25.*
15. Darrah J, Watkins B, Chen L, Bonin C. Effects of conductive education intervention for children with a diagnosis of cerebral palsy: an AACPDM evidence report. *Dev Med Child Neurol.* 2004;46:187-203.
16. Charles J, Gordon AM. A critical review of constraint-induced movement therapy and forced use in children with hemiplegia. *Neural Plasticity.* 2005;12(2-3):245-261.
17. Autti-Rämö I, Suoranta J, Antilla H, Malmivaara A, Makela M. Effectiveness of upper and lower limb casting and orthoses in children with cerebral palsy: an overview of the review articles. *Am J Phys Med Rehabil.* 2006;85(1):89-103.
18. *Morris C. A review of the efficacy of lower-limb orthoses used for cerebral palsy. Dev Med Child Neurol. 2002;44:205-211.*
19. Hur JJ. Review of research on therapeutic intervention for children with cerebral palsy. *Acta Neurol Scand.* 1995;91:423-432.
20. Teplicky R, Law M, Russell D. The effectiveness of casts, orthoses, and splints for children with neurological disorders. *Inf Young Child.* 2002;15(1):42-50.
21. Blauw-Hospers CH, Hadders-Algra M. A systematic review of the effects of early intervention on motor development. *Dev Med Child Neurol.* 2005;47:421-432.
22. Brown GT, Burns SA. The efficacy of neurodevelopmental treatment in paediatrics: a systematic review. *Br J Occup Ther.* 2001;64:235-244.
23. Butler C, Darrah J. Effects of neurodevelopmental treatment (NDT) for cerebral palsy: an AACPDM evidence report. *Dev Med Child Neurol.* 2001;43:778-790.
24. LaForme Fiss AC, Effgen SK. Outcomes for young children with disabilities associated with the use of partial body weight supported treadmill training: an evidence based review. *Phys Ther Rev.* 2006;11:179-189.
25. Leong B. Critical review of passive muscle stretch: implications for the treatment of children in vegetative and minimally conscious states. *Brain Inj.* 2002;16:169-183.
26. Pin T, Dyke P, Chan M. The effectiveness of passive stretching in children with cerebral palsy. *Dev Med Child Neurol.* 2006;48:855-862.
27. Darrah J, Fan JSW, Chen LC, Nunweiler J, Watkins B. Review of the effects of progressive resisted muscle strengthening in children with cerebral palsy: a clinical consensus exercise. *Pediatr Phys Ther.* 1997;9:12-17.
28. Dodd KJ, Taylor NF, Damiano DL. A systematic review of the effectiveness of strength-training programs for people with cerebral palsy. *Arch Phys Med Rehabil.* 2002;83:1157-1164.
29. Pin TW. Effectiveness of static weight-bearing exercises in children with cerebral palsy. *Pediatr Phys Ther.* 2007;19:62-73.

30. LaForme Fiss AC, Effgen SK. Use of groups in pediatric physical therapy: survey of current practices. *Pediatr Phys Ther.* 2007;19:154-159.
31. Rainforth B, York-Barr J. *Collaborative Teams for Students With Severe Disabilities: Integrating Therapy and Educational Services.* 2nd ed. Baltimore, MD: Paul H. Brookes; 1997.
32. McEwen IR, Shelden ML. Pediatric therapy in the 1990s: the demise of the educational versus medical dichotomy. In: McEwen IR, ed. *Occupational and Physical Therapy in Educational Environments.* Binghamton, NY: Haworth Press; 1995:33-45.
33. Adolph KE, Vereijken B, Shrout PE. What changes in infant walking and why. *Child Dev.* 2003;74:475-497.
34. Kleim JA. III STEP: a basic scientist's perspective. *Phys Ther. 2006;86:614-617.*
35. American Physical Therapy Association Code of Ethics (HOD S06-00-12-23). Alexandria, VA: American Physical Therapy Association; 2000. http://www.apta.org/AM/Template.cfm?Section=Core_Documents1&Template=/CM/HTMLDisplay.cfm&ContentID=25854. Accessed November 10, 2007.
36. Rainforth B. Analysis of physical therapy practice acts: implications for role release in educational environments. *Pediatr Phys Ther.* 1997;9:54-61.
37. Nolan KW, Mannato L, Wilding GE. Integrated models of pediatric physical and occupational therapy: regional practice and related outcomes. *Pediatr Phys Ther.* 2004;16:121-128.
38. Larin HM. Motor learning: theories and strategies for the practitioner. In: Campbell SK, Vander Linden DW, Palisano RJ, eds. *Physical Therapy for Children.* 3rd ed. St Louis, MO: Sanders Elsevier; 2006:131-160.
39. Kaminker MK, Chiarello LA, Chiarini Smith JA. Decision making for physical therapy service delivery in schools: a nationwide analysis by geographic region. *Pediatr Phys Ther.* 2006;18:204-213.

10
Assistive Technology

Amanda Porter, PT, MPT, and Maria Jones, PT, PhD, ATP

A major role of physical therapists, especially those who work with infants, toddlers, and children with severe disabilities, is identifying, recommending, and/or providing assistive technology devices and services. Many children need mobility devices, computers, communication devices, environmental modifications, and other technology to achieve their developmental and educational goals or participate in educational and other natural environments. All technology is not sophisticated and expensive; something as simple as a pencil holder or tape to hold a worksheet on a desk is assistive technology.

What does IDEA say about assistive technology?

Sec. 303.13 of Part C includes assistive technology as one of the early intervention services that states are required to provide to meet the developmental needs of infants and toddlers with disabilities, as identified by the individualized family service plan. Sec. 300.105 of Part B states:

> *(a) Each public agency shall ensure that assistive technology devices or assistive technology services, or both, as those terms are defined in Secs. 300.5-300.6, are made available to a child with a disability if required as part of the child's—*
> *(1) Special education under Sec. 300.39;*
> *(2) Related services under Sec. 300.34; or*
> *(3) Supplementary aides and services under Sec. 300.42 and 300.114(a)(2)(ii).*

This means that schools will make assistive technology devices and services available, if students need them as part of special education, related services, or as a supplementary aid or service in a general education classroom.

What are the definitions of assistive technology devices and services?

Sec. 303.12(1)(i) of Part C defines an assistive technology device as:

> *... any item, piece of equipment, or product system, whether acquired commercially off the shelf, modified, or customized, that is used to increase, maintain, or improve the functional capabilities of an infant or toddler with a disability. The term does not include a medical device that is surgically implanted, including cochlear implants, or the optimization (e.g., mapping) or the maintenance or replacement of that device.*

Similarly, Sec. 300.5 of Part B defines an assistive technology device as:

> *… any item, piece of equipment, or product system, whether acquired commercially off the shelf, modified, or customized, that is used to increase, maintain, or improve the functional capabilities of children with disabilities. The term does not include a medical device that is surgically implanted, or the replacement of such device.*

The definition of assistive technology service is included in both Part C and Part B and covers many services that physical therapists provide. Sec. 303.13(b)(1)(ii)(a-f) of Part C for and Sec. 300.6 of Part B define assistive technology service as:

> *… any service that directly assists an infant or toddler or a child with a disability in the selection, acquisition, or use of an assistive technology device. The term includes—*
>
> *(a) The evaluation of the needs of an infant or toddlers or a child with a disability, including a functional evaluation of the infant or toddler or child in the child's customary environment;*
>
> *(b) Purchasing, leasing, or otherwise providing for the acquisition of assistive technology devices by infants or toddler or children with disabilities;*
>
> *(c) Selecting, designing, fitting, customizing, adapting, applying, maintaining, repairing, or replacing assistive technology devices;*
>
> *(d) Coordinating and using other therapies, interventions, or services with assistive technology devices, such as those associated with existing education and rehabilitation plans and programs;*
>
> *(e) Training or technical assistance for an infant or toddler or a child with a disability or, if appropriate, that child's family; and*
>
> *(f) Training or technical assistance for professionals (including individuals providing education and rehabilitation services), employers, or other individuals who provide services to, employ, or are otherwise substantially involved in the major life functions of infant and toddler or children with disabilities.*

Do early intervention programs and school districts have to address infants', toddlers', or students' needs for assistive technology?

Yes, when teams are developing an individualized family service plan (IFSP), the team must determine the early intervention services that are necessary to meet the unique needs of the child and the family to achieve the identified results or outcomes (Sec. 303.344). For children receiving services under Part B, the IEP team must take into consideration the special factors listed in Sec. 300.324, which include consideration of the (1) positive behavioral interventions and supports and other strategies to address behavior that impede the children's learning or that of others; (2) language needs of the child for children with limited English proficiency; (3) Braille instruction or use of Braille for children who are blind or visually impaired; (4) communication needs and opportunities for direct communications with peers and professional personnel in the child's language and communication mode for children who are deaf or hard or hearing, and (5) assistive technology devices and services needs of children. More specifically, Sec. 300.324(a)(2)(v) says that the IEP shall "consider whether the child needs assistive technology devices and services." The manner in which early intervention services and consideration of special factors, including assistive technology, are documented on IFSP and IEP forms varies from state to state. Physical therapists should become familiar with state forms, policies, and procedures to ensure documentation is completed appropriately.

What happens when team members do not agree about assistive technology?

Sometimes team members do not agree with decisions about assistive technology devices and services or have questions about it. Table 10-1 summarizes court decisions, letters of inquiry, and policy interpretations related to assistive technology, which can help clarify the process and the intent of the law. See the introduction to Section III of this book for an overview of due process decisions at state and federal levels and a brief overview of the United States judicial organizational structure.

Table 10-1. Assistive Technology Court Decisions, Letters of Inquiry, and Policy Interpretation[a]

Federal Court of Appeals

Case	Citation	Jurisdiction	Issue	Comments
Sherman and Nishanian ex rel. Nishanian v. Mamaroneck Union Free Sch. Dist.	39 IDELR 181	2003 appeal from the United States District Court, Southern District of New York	FAPE	An advanced calculator was not required because the older model calculated the answer requiring the student to perform each step of the problem, whereas the new calculator would do the entire problem with the push of a button.

Federal District Court

Case	Citation	Jurisdiction	Issue	Comments
A.S. and W.S. ex rel. Mr. and Mrs. W.S. v. Trumbull Bd. of Educ.	45 IDELR 40	D. Ct. 2006	Provision of AT	Even though the parents requested a specific reading program, the school was implementing appropriate AT and methodologies that benefited the student.
Eric H. by John and Janet H. v. Methacton Sch. Dist.	38 IDELR 182	E.D. Penn 2003	Provision of AT	Video teleconferencing was not necessary to achieve social and behavioral objectives because opportunities to address those needs existed during school attendance.
Kevin T. v. Elmhurst Community Sch. Dist. No. 205	36 IDELR 153	N.D. Ill. 2002	Consideration of AT	District violated provisions of IDEA by failing to consider the student's need for assistive technology.
Board of Education of Harford County vs. Bauer	33 IDELR 267	D. Md. 2000	Location of AT services	District must provide assistive technology for a student who was privately placed.
East Penn School District vs. Scott B	29 IDELR 1058	E.D. Penn. 1999	Compensatory AT services	Compensatory AT devices and services were required because a student's IEP was substantially flawed.

State Courts

Case	Citation	Jurisdiction	Issue	Comments
Vega ex Rel. Maestre vs. Dept of Education	33 IDELR 246	PR Court of Appeals 2000	Provision of AT	District required to provide a wheelchair because student's age and use of a wheelchair outside of school was not grounds for denying purchase.
In Re: The Adoption of Amendments to N.J.A.C. 6:28-2.10, 3.6 and 4.3	27 IDELR 27	New Jersey Superior Court, Appellate Division	AT definition	Court ruled that a New Jersey state special education regulation was invalid because it required the inclusion of "specialized equipment and materials" in IEP, but failed to define the term, and made it impossible to determine whether the term included assistive technology devices as defined by IDEA and the Technology-Related Assistance for Individuals with Disabilities Act.

State Education Agencies (SEA)

Case	Citation	Jurisdiction	Issue	Comments
Los Angeles Unified School District	46 IDELR 232	SEA CA 2006	Provision of AT	District was not obligated to provide top-of-the-line equipment, even if available.
Collier County Sch. Bd.	44 IDELR 80	SEA FL 2005	Provision of AT	District was not required to provide the device the family requested because the district offered devices that would further the student's IEP goals.
Gaylord Community Schs	40 IDELR 224	SEA MI 2003	Provision of AT	District did not have to provide and pay for oxygen and oxygen tanks but was responsible for related equipment (eg portable cart and oxygen monitoring equipment).
Malden Pub. Schs.	39 IDELR 275	SEA MA 2003	Provision of AT	District required to reimburse the costs of an FM loop system because of failure to ensure FM training device was properly functioning.
Jefferson County Sch. Dist. R-1	39 IDELR 119	SEA CO 2003	Provision of AT	District did not have to provide at-home computer because student could not show his academic performance would suffer without the device.
El Paso Indep. Sch. Dist.	38 IDELR 26	SEA TX 2002	Provision of AT	District required to provide compensatory training because although student received assistive technology, he was unable to use the equipment without training.
Houston Indep. Sch. Dist.	36 IDELR 286	SEA TX 2002	Provision of AT FAPE	Although the student could clearly benefit from a laptop computer with voice recognition capabilities for use at school and home, she did not need the assistive technology device to receive an FAPE.
Laredo Indep. Sch. Dist.	36 IDELR 171	SEA TX 2002	Provision of AT FAPE	District did not have to provide laptop computer and an audio books program because student need was not evident. The student had access to numerous assistive technology devices and received 1:1 support from 2 tutors.
Brandywine Pub. Schs.	35 IDELR 81	SEA MI 2001	Provision of AT FAPE	Because district failed to provide an adapted toilet seat and a specially designed computer keyboard and accompanying software as indicated in IEP, student was not receiving FAPE and was entitled to services, as originally specified.
Fort Bend Indep. Sch. Dist.	34 IDELR 246	SEA TX 2001	Provision of AT LRE	District was not required to provide a computer program for language skills, which may have been the best available technology, because IEP offered educational benefit in the LRE.
Jefferson County Sch. Dist. R-1	34 IDELR 212	SEA CO 2001	Provision of AT FAPE	District not required to provide a home computer because student did not require computer to make educational progress.
Houston Indep. Sch. Dist.	34 IDELR 165	SEA TX 2000	Provision of AT FAPE	District provided appropriate notice of assistive technology evaluation and even though parents failed to consent, the district did not deny FAPE. District not required to use standardized tests in conducting its evaluation.
Board of Educ. of the City Sch. Dist. of the City of NY.	34 IDELR 163	SEA NY 2000	Provision of AT LRE	District did not have to reimburse parents for private school tuition because they provided the appropriate assistive technology and instructed student on use of the devices.

State Education Agencies (SEA) (continued)

Case	Citation	Jurisdiction	Issue	Comments
Board of Educ. of the Mamaroneck Union Free Sch. Dist.	34 IDELR 107	SEA NY 2000	Provision of AT FAPE	District did not have to provide a higher functioning calculator because AT device offered by the district provided the student with FAPE and student had grade-appropriate math skills with the use of device.
Progreso Indep. Sch. Dist	34 IDELR 103	SEA TX 2000	Provision of AT FAPE	District did not have to provide hearing aid because it was not required for the student to benefit from his education.
Tuscaloosa City Bd. of Educ.	34 IDELR 83	SEA AL 2000	Provision of AT FAPE	District did not have to provide a student with a different augmentative communication device, as requested by the student's mother. Judge ruled that the student's use of an augmentative communication device provided FAPE and a "basic floor of opportunity," allowing him to make progress.
East Whittier City Elementary Sch. Dist.	34 IDELR 49	SEA CA 2000	Provision of AT	District did not have to provide a home laptop computer because even though the student missed school frequently due to a chronic condition, the desktop computers and direct instruction she received while at school were sufficient to properly implement the IEP.
Greater Albany Pub. Sch. Dist.	32 IDELR 157	SEA OR 1999	Provision of AT	District appropriately discontinued assistive technology from the IEP because the student was making adequate progress without the technology.
School District of the City of Beacon	30 IDELR 937	SEA NY 1999	Reimbursement	District did not have to reimburse family for a communication device because other means of communication were in place.
Dalles School District	30 IDELR 631	SEA OR 1998	Provision of AT	Delay in instructional assistant's understanding the use of communication device did not deny FAPE because multiple means of communication were available.
Ankeny Community Sch. Dist.	30 IDELR 451	SEA IA 1999	Provision of AT	District's choice of signing methodology was appropriate and compatible with the parent's preferred system. No indication that student was denied benefit from using district's methodology.
In Re: Student with a Disability	29 IDELR 809	SEA DE 1998	Provision of AT FAPE	FAPE denied when IEP that called for written language expression tutoring and appropriate assistive technology was not provided.
East Allegheny Sch. Dist.	29 IDELR 662	SEA PA 1998	Provision of AT FAPE	FAPE denied when district failed to provide another communication device despite knowing of parents' dissatisfaction and having recommendations from the district's assistive technology specialist for a different device. District ordered to provide the specific device, along with training to learn to use the device.
Upper Darby Sch. Dist.	26 IDELR 1183	SEA PA 1997	Provision of AT FAPE	District denied FAPE when it proposed an inadequate IEP by failing to provide AT despite considerable evidence of the need for a portable computer.
Glendale Union High Sch. Dist	26 IDELR 243	SEA AZ 1997	Provision of AT	District required to provide on-site interpreter services to a student voluntarily enrolled in a parochial school.
Highland Local Sch. Dist.	26 IDELR 224	SEA OH 1997	Provision of AT	District provided adequate communication goals, instruction in a variety of modalities, and staff training, including use of an augmentative communication device with auditory output.

State Education Agencies (SEA) (continued)

Case	Citation	Jurisdiction	Issue	Comments
Silsbee Indep. Sch. Dist.	25 IDELR 1023	SEA TX 1997	Provision of AT Definition of AT	District required to provide oxygen tanks as assistive technology to ensure the student was able to attend school.
Austin Indep. Sch. Dist.	25 IDELR 875	SEA TX 1997	Provision of AT	District not obligated to provide an alternate reading program because an appropriate reading program was in place and student was making progress with current program.
Bd. of Educ. of Smithtown Central Sch. Dist.	22 IDELR 818	SEA NY 1995	Provision of AT	District not required to use a frequency modulated auditory trainer (FM trainer) in the classroom because student made academic progress and social gains without the use of an FM trainer during the previous school year.
In re Child with a Disability	21 IDELR 749	SEA CT 1994	Provision of AT FAPE	After a student's computer disappeared, replacement of the computer that served as an augmentative communication device with a different type of communication device did not deny FAPE as both devices provided educational benefit.
Maynard Sch. Dist.	20 IDELR 394	SEA AR 1993	Environmental access	As a recipient of federal assistance under the IDEA, the state is responsible to ensure that all public agencies involved in the education of children with disabilities meet the requirements for removal of architectural barriers.
Greenwood County Sch. Dist. #52	19 IDELR 355	SEA SC 1992	Provision of AT	District required to purchase communication device, to incorporate device into IEP, and to provide opportunity for use because evidence existed that student would benefit from such a device and could not receive educational benefit without it.
Davis Sch. Dist.	18 IDELR 696	SEA UT 1992	Provision of AT	District required to consult with the state's department of education and to select, in cooperation with the parents, an appropriate assistive device for school bus loading and unloading.

Federal Agencies (OSEP, OSERS, OCR)

Case	Citation	Jurisdiction	Issue	Comments
Seminole County (FL) Sch. Dist.	46 IDELR 262	OCR 2006	Section 504 of ADA	District did not violate Section 504 or the ADA when it failed to honor a parent's request to regularly reprogram a student's communication device for increased interaction with students and staff.
Cuyahoga Falls (OH) City Sch. Dist.	43 IDELR 226	OCR 2004	Provision of AT/FAPE	Student was not denied FAPE because IEP required provision of a Gemini computer and adaptive feeding equipment, which district provided along with appropriate replacements when specified items were unavailable.
Fayette County (KY) Sch. Dist.	40 IDELR 130	OCR 2003	Provision of AT	Parent's claim that the district failed to appropriately implement student's 504 plan by providing a laptop computer, adaptive physical education, and occupational therapy was rejected because the 504 plan did not require use of such devices and/or services.
Letter to Goodman	4 ECLPR 497	OSEP 2003	Provision of AT	OSEP clarified that assistive technology devices and services are included as early intervention services under Part C of the IDEA.

Federal Agencies (OSEP, OSERS, OCR) (continued)

Case	Citation	Jurisdiction	Issue	Comments
Issaquah (WA) Sch. Dist. No. 411	40 IDELR 53	OCR 2003	Provision of AT FAPE	Parent's allegation that a district violated FAPE because the district was delayed in providing a rocking chair and failed to provide an FM system was rejected. The district provided the rocking chair 2 days into the student's educational program and neither student nor district believed an FM system was needed.
Benicia (California) Unified School District	30 IDELR 900	OCR 1998	Provision of AT	District agreed to provide an audiologist, back-up interpreter, and a working sound field system when parents alleged discrimination.
Letter to Hutcheson	30 IDELR 708	OSEP 1998	Provision of AT	Both state and local educational agencies have obligations related to provision of AT devices and services.
Letter to Goodman	30 IDELR 611	OSEP 1998	Location of AT	Equipment funded under Part B can be used by student in state vocational rehabilitation programs and ownership can be transferred if no longer needed by the district.
Letter from anonymous	29 IDELR 1089	OSEP 1997	Provision of AT	Parent requested assistance in obtaining a computer for her child. Process for obtaining device for FAPE clarified.
Hancock (NY) Central Sch. Dist	29 IDELR 916	OCR 1998	Provisions of AT Discrimination	District did not discriminate against a student by failing to connect communication device to computer because no evidence existed for student's use of the communication device to complete assignments.
Letter to Culbreath	25 IDELR 1212	OSEP 1997	Provision of AT	State law governs who is liable for the damage or loss of publicly-owned AT devices provided as a part of FAPE that are damaged due to negligence or abuse, or are lost or stolen. Such state laws must be consistent with Part B and the right to a FAPE and districts can not charge parents for normal use and wear and tear of the devices.
Letter to Anonymous	24 IDELR 854	OSEP 1996		If an IEP team determines a student requires AT services/devices to receive FAPE, then the specific devices and services must be identified in the child's IEP. The structure of the IEP document, including whether the IEP must contain a section addressing assistive technology, falls within the public agency's discretion.
Letter to Anonymous	24 IDELR 388	OSEP 1996	Provision of AT	Generally, a public agency is not required to provide an AT device/service for a student if that student would require the device or service regardless of whether he or she attended school. However, if the student requires the device or service to receive FAPE, then it must be provided.
Letter to Fisher	23 IDELR 565	OSEP 1995	AT evaluation	A parent can request an independent evaluation to determine the need for AT where the school neglects to evaluate the student for assistive technology needs or when the parent disagrees with the school's evaluation.
Letter to Naon	22 IDELR 888	OSEP 1995	Provision of AT	Public agency must ensure AT devices and services necessary for FAPE are provided. The IEP team determines whether AT devices and services are needed.

Federal Agencies (OSEP, OSERS, OCR) (continued)

Case	Citation	Jurisdiction	Issue	Comments
Letter to Bachus	22 IDELR 629	OSEP 1995	Provision of AT	If a child with a disability requires eyeglasses to receive FAPE and the child's IEP specifies the need for eyeglasses, then the public agency must provide them at no cost to the parents and could seek funds from outside of the agency to do so.
Letter to Galloway	22 IDELR 373	OSEP 1994	Provision of AT	If the IEP indicates the need for an AT device such as a hearing aid as part of special education, then district must provide the device at no cost to the parents. State law, regulation, and policy would determine whether the home school district or the state school for the deaf would be responsible for payment.
Letter to Anonymous	21 IDELR 1126	OSEP 1993	Provision of AT	Audiology services and AT must be provided only if the services are necessary to meet the developmental needs of the child and the needs of his or her family on the IFSP.
Letter to Anonymous	21 IDELR 1057	OSEP 1994	Provision of AT	Districts should assume responsibility to repair a family-owned AT device because the district is responsible for providing services and devices in the IEP, and without the use of the family-owned device, the district would have to provide and maintain the device.
Letter to Anonymous	21 IDELR 745	OSEP 1994	Provision of AT	Provision of a device/service in a parentally-placed private school is permitted, if the district's implementation of the equitable participation requirement includes the provision of such device/services.
Letter to Seiler	20 IDELR 1216	OSEP 1993	Definition of AT	A hearing aid is considered a covered device under the definition of "assistive technology device."
Letter to Cohen	19 IDELR 278	OSEP 1992	Funding for AT	State and local educational agencies may access alternative funding to defray the costs of providing AT devices and services only if use does not result in a reduction of benefits or in an alteration of eligibility.
Letter to Lambert	18 IDELR 1039	OSEP 1992	Definition of AT	A calculator could fit the definition of an assistive technology device under Part B.
Letter to Anonymous	18 IDELR 1037	OSEP 1992	Provision of AT	Parents can request an impartial due process hearing, or file a complaint with the state educational agency if they believe denial of FM system is preventing FAPE.
Letter to Anonymous	18 IDELR 627	OSEP 1991	Provision of AT FAPE	If an IEP team determines that a child needs access to an AT device at home for FAPE, then district must provide the device for home use to implement the IEP.

[a]The table is organized by jurisdiction, or level of authority, and then entries are listed in chronological order (starting with most recent) within each level or section. Physical therapists should locate and read decisions in their entirety before applying them to a new scenario or situation. Citations to the IDELR (Individuals with Disabilities Education Law Report),8 formerly the EHLR (Education of the Handicapped Law Report),9 refer to a loose leaf publication from the LRP Publishing Company. All of the documents referenced in the table are public information and can be obtained through multiple avenues via the Internet or as hard copies. Assistance in locating the documents can be obtained in many state departments of education, special education regional resource centers, larger university education or law libraries, and larger law firms specializing in education law.

Do all infants or toddlers with an IFSP or students with an IEP require an assistive technology evaluation to determine the need for devices and/or services?

No. A formal assistive technology evaluation is not required for every infant and toddler with an IFSP or every student with an IEP. Section 303.344 of Part C says that the IFSP must include the early intervention services that are necessary to meet the unique needs of the child and the family to achieve the results or outcomes. Sec. 300.324(a)(2)(v) of Part B, however, says that the IEP team shall "consider whether the child needs assistive technology devices and services." The assistive technology services may include an evaluation.

What is the difference between consideration and evaluation?

Consideration is a process that involves brief discussion and examination of assistive technology options, which frequently occurs during the IEP meeting and results in 1 of 4 decisions: (1) current interventions and strategies are working and nothing new, including assistive technology, is needed; (2) assistive technology is already being used and is working; (3) a student requires trials with new assistive technology; or (4) the team needs to gather more information to make a decision, thus moving on to an evaluation.[1] Evaluation requires more time and involves gathering additional and often new information about the student's abilities and difficulties, the demands of the educational environments, and the tasks required in those environments.

Do teams have to reconsider the need for assistive technology when an IFSP or IEP is reviewed and modified?

Yes. According to Sec. 303.342(b)(ii) of Part C, the IFSP team must determine whether modification or review of the outcomes or services, including assistive technology, are necessary when reviewing and/or modifying the IFSP. Similarly, the IEP team must reconsider the special factors, including assistive technology, when reviewing the IEP (Sec. 300.324[b][2]).

Who is qualified to do an assistive technology evaluation?

Professionals in early intervention, special education, and related services can be qualified to provide assistive technology evaluations. Evaluations should include a team of professionals and should be performed by professionals who are knowledgeable about assistive technology. As a general rule, the team should include: (1) a person knowledgeable about the infant or toddler or student (most likely the student and/or parents); (2) a person knowledgeable in the area of cognitive development and/or curriculum (eg, early childhood educator or special education teacher); (3) a person knowledgeable in the area of language/communication (eg, speech/language pathologist); (4) a person knowledgeable about motor activities and requirements (eg, occupational therapist or physical therapist); and (5) a person who can authorize use of the school district's resources (eg, administrator).[1] The make-up of the team will vary based on the infant's, toddler's, or student's unique needs.

Where should assistive technology devices and services be documented in the IFSP or IEP?

Although individual state and early intervention program IFSP forms vary, as do state and district IEP forms, assistive technology can be documented in many ways. Under Part C, assistive technology should be included as an early intervention service when it is necessary to assist the child in achieving identified outcomes. For children receiving services under Part B, assistive technology can be included as part of special education, as a related service, and/or as a supplementary aid and service. Physical therapists should become familiar with state, early intervention program, and district policies and procedures for documenting assistive technology devices and services in the IFSP or IEP.

Can an early intervention program or school district ask an IFSP or IEP team not to list assistive technology on an IFSP/IEP because the program or school district will have to pay for it?

No. An early intervention program or a school district cannot "presumptively deny" assistive technology to infants, toddlers, or students with disabilities without first determining whether the child requires an assistive technology device or service to achieve IFSP outcomes or obtain a "free and appropriate public education" (FAPE). Early intervention programs should determine the need for assistive technology on an individual basis in conjunction with the development of the infant's or toddler's IFSP. Similarly, school districts must determine the need for assistive technology on an individual basis in conjunction with the development of the student's IEP.[2] Physical therapists and other professionals play a key role in assessing infants', toddlers', and students' needs for assistive technology and recommending appropriate devices and/or services that enable children with disabilities to achieve outcomes and benefit from the educational process. Physical therapists, as a member of IFSP and IEP teams, should not hesitate to make assistive technology recommendations because of cost. Physical therapists can play an important role in assisting the early intervention program, school, and family to identify other funding sources available to the student with disabilities.[3]

Can an early intervention program or school district use outside funding sources to pay for assistive technology as part of an IFSP/IEP?

Yes. As stated in Part C, Sec. 303.12(b)(1)(ii)(b), early intervention programs can purchase, lease, or otherwise provide for the acquisition of assistive technology. Nothing in Parts C or B prevent an early intervention program or school district from pursuing funding from outside sources, such as Medicaid or other public funding sources or private insurance, as long as the equipment is provided at no cost to the infant, toddler, or student or the parents.[4] Part C, Sec. 303.520, specifically addresses policies related to use of insurance or public benefits for payment of services for infants, toddlers, and their families. Part B, Sec. 300.154, addresses methods for ensuring services, including use of public benefits and insurance to pay for services, including assistive technology, necessary to provide an FAPE.

Can a school district refuse to let students take home school-purchased assistive technology?

No. Schools cannot refuse to let students use equipment at home if it is required to implement the IEP. The student's IEP should include a specific statement of assistive technology devices or services the student requires to receive an FAPE, including the nature and amount of such services.[5] A student's education does not stop at the end of the school day. Students are expected use and further refine information and skills learned in school outside the school setting. Sec. 300.105(b) says:

> *On a case-by-case basis, the use of school-purchased assistive technology devices in a child's home or in other settings is required if the child's IEP team determines that the child needs access to those devices in order to receive FAPE.*

Who owns assistive technology purchased by the early intervention program or school?

The assistive technology is the property of the early intervention program or school, just as textbooks and band instruments that a school purchases belong to the school. A response to a comment prior to the reauthorization of IDEA 1997 (PL 105-17) said:

> *...while ownership of the devices in these circumstances (devices purchased by the school) would remain with the public agency, State law, rather than Part B, generally would determine whether parent's are liable for the loss, theft, or damage due to negligence or misuse of publicly owned equipment used at home or in other settings in accordance with the IEP.*

What should an early intervention program or school district do if parents have recommendations for assistive technology from an outside evaluator and ask the early intervention program or school district to purchase the technology, but the rest of the IFSP or IEP team does not believe the assistive technology is needed?

Under Part B, school districts are not required to implement all the recommendations provided by the independent evaluator, but according to Sec. 300.502(c)(1):

> *If the parent obtains an independent educational evaluation at public expense or shares with the public agency an evaluation obtained at private expense, the results of the evaluation must be considered by the public agency, if it meets agency criteria, in any decision made with respect to the provision of FAPE to the child.*

If the IEP team can show, on an individual basis, using IDEA Part B procedures for evaluation, IEP development, and placement, that the student does not require the recommended assistive technology to receive an FAPE, then the district does not have to provide the assistive technology. The evaluation should assess a student's functional abilities with and without assistive technology in the student's educational environment(s).[6] Similar procedures would be necessary for IFSP teams to determine whether an infant or toddler required assistive technology to achieve identified outcomes.

If an infant, toddler, or student owns equipment needed to accomplish IFSP or IEP outcomes/goals, but the equipment breaks and the family cannot pay for repair, does the early intervention program or school have any responsibility to repair the equipment?

If a family-owned assistive technology device becomes unavailable for any reason, the early intervention program or school must continue to implement the IFSP or IEP, providing either a substitute device or reviewing the IFSP or IEP with all team members to determine if the device still is needed.[6] It may be appropriate for the early intervention program or school district to assume responsibility for repairing the device, because it would be responsible for the device if it is specified as part of the IFSP or IEP.

If students need access to altered instructional materials, what are the provisions for ensuring access to those materials?

> *For students who are blind and cannot see the words or images on a page, cannot hold a book or turn its pages, cannot decode the text or cannot comprehend the syntax that supports the written word may each experience different challenges, and they may each require different supports to extract meaning from information that is "book bound."*[7]

For these students, various types of altered formats, including Braille translation, large-print books, books on tape, or electronic books may be necessary. Each state has the option of adopting the National Instructional Materials Accessibility Standards (NIMAS), which were added into IDEA 2004. Regardless of whether or not states adopt NIMAS, Sec. 300.172(b)(4) says, "the SEA must ensure that all public agencies take all reasonable steps to provide instructional materials in accessible formats to children with disabilities who need those instructional materials at the same time as other children receive instructional materials." Because many students who require altered instructional materials will use assistive technology, Sec. 300.172(d) says, "the state educational agency, to the maximum extent possible, shall work collaboratively with the State agency responsible for assistive technology programs."

States are currently developing procedures whereby local school districts and service providers can obtain accessible instructional materials for students, so physical therapists should become familiar with the state and local district procedures to ensure students get the materials they need at the same time as other students.

SUMMARY

The 1997 amendments of IDEA strengthened the requirement for IEP and IFSP teams to consider infants', toddlers', and students' needs for assistive technology devices and services, and IDEA 2004 continues to support the importance of considering assistive technology for every infant, toddler, and student, and it expanded consideration to include when an IFSP or IEP is reviewed and modified. If the IFSP team determines that infants or toddlers need assistive technology as an early intervention service, the early intervention program must make the technology available. Similarly, if an IEP team determines that a student needs assistive technology as special education, a related service, or a supplementary aid and service, the district must make the technology available to the student. Early intervention programs and school districts may pay for the assistive technology, but also may use other available resources, such as third-party payers, as long as infant, toddler, student, or parents do not incur costs associated with the purchase of the device. Along with the continued provisions for assistive technology, IDEA 2004 emphasizes the importance of providing accessible instructional materials to students in a timely manner.

REFERENCES

1. Reed P, Lahm E, eds. *Assessing Student's Needs for Assistive Technology.* Oshkosh, WI: Wisconsin Assistive Technology Initiative; 2004.
2. Schrag JA. Letter to Goodman, 16 Education for the Handicapped Law Reporter (EHLR) 1317 (1990).
3. Palette HP, Hofmann A, VanBiervliet A. The professional's role in obtaining funding for assistive technology for infants and toddlers with disabilities. *Teaching Except Child.* 1994;Spring;22-28.
4. Schrag JA. Letter to Spann, 20 Individuals With Disabilities Education Law Report (IDELR) 627 (1993).
5. Schrag JA. Letter to Anonymous, 18 Individuals With Disabilities Education Law Report (IDELR) 627 (1991).
6. Hehir T. Letter to Anonymous, 21 Individuals With Disabilities Education Law Report (IDELR) 1057 (1994).
7. National Instructional Materials Accessibility Standards Web site. The need for flexible alternatives to print. http://nimas.cast.org/about/index.html. Accessed July 31, 2007.
8. Individuals With Disabilities Education Law Report. West Palm Beach, FL: LRP Publications.
9. Education of the Handicapped Law Report. West Palm Beach, FL: LRP Publications.

11
Extended School Year Services

Sandra Arnold, PT, PhD

Extended school year (ESY) services are special education and related services that are provided for a student with a disability beyond the normal school year in accordance with the student's IEP, at no cost to the student's parents, and that meet the standards of the state education agency (Sec. 300.10).[1] A school district may not limit ESY services to children with particular categories of disabilities, or unilaterally limit the type, amount, or duration of those services (Sec. 300.106[a][3]). ESY services usually take place during the summer, but could occur at other times if districts have major breaks at other times of the year. Each school district usually has specific ESY policies.

Can all students receive extended school year services?

No. The determination of whether a student requires ESY is made on an individual basis. According to Sec. 300.106(a)(2):

> *Extended school year services must be provided only if a child's IEP team determines, on an individual basis, in accordance with Secs. 300.320-300.324, that the services are necessary for the provision of FAPE to the child.*

Generally, if the IEP team determines that the student will experience loss of skills or regression during the break from school, which the student will not recoup within a reasonable time after returning to school, then ESY services should be made available to the student. Although IDEA regulations do not directly address the terms "regression" and "recoupment," case laws have interpreted regression to mean that the decline in knowledge and skills that can result from an interruption in education and recoupment to mean the amount of time it takes to regain the prior level of functioning, as determined by the individual IEP team.[2,3] The team decides if the skills the student learned during the school year will be significantly or substantially jeopardized if the student is not provided educational programming during the summer months or other major break.[2]

Are regression and recoupment the only considerations for ESY services?

No. The need for ESY services for each individual student is a mutltifactoral determination.[4] Factors to be considered include, but are not limited to, the nature and extent of the student's disability, the student's rate of progress, the student's need for interaction with peers without disabilities, the degree of regression in the past, availability of alternative resources, the parent's ability to provide educational structure at home, emerging skills and breakthrough opportunities (as when the child is on the brink of beginning to walk), and predictive data based on opinion of professionals.[2-4]

When should ESY services be determined?

Determination of ESY service for a student should be made early enough in the year to allow the parents adequate time to exercise their right to administrative review or appeal in a timely fashion if the rest of the team decides a student does not need ESY and the parents disagree.[2,3] Usually ESY services are planned during the month of April.

Can a physical therapist decide if a student is eligible for ESY services?

No. Physical therapists cannot independently make decisions about service delivery for students. The IEP team, of which the physical therapist should be a part, determines if a student is eligible for ESY services. The physical therapist can provide information to assist team members in making an educated decision about a student's need for ESY services.

Should ESY services be provided to a student to maximize the student's education?

No. Although IDEA provides for a free and appropriate public education, it does not guarantee the best possible education.[1] ESY services cannot be provided just for the purpose of maximizing a student's educational opportunities. Similarly, it is not enough that the student will regress if the student does not receive educational programming over a break. Students in general education lose some skills or knowledge during the summer. The amount of regression must be significant or substantial. IDEA cannot be used to fund a level of educational programming that exceeds the level of benefit to which general education students are entitled.[5]

Can students in private schools receive ESY services?

Yes. Students with disabilities who have been placed in private schools, and are designated by the local education agency (LEA) to receive special education and related services, retain all of the rights under IDEA, including the right to ESY services (Secs. 300.132, 300.138, 300.146, 300.148). Private schools, however, are not responsible for ensuring a FAPE and therefore are not obligated to offer ESY services. The state education agency is obligated to provide alternative placements for the summer months or other major breaks if a private school chooses not to provide ESY for an eligible student.

Can states and/or districts categorically deny ESY services to students with certain characteristics or categories of disabilities?

No. Just as students can not be categorically placed in classrooms or programs (see Chapter 5), students cannot be categorically denied ESY services.[1] To categorically deny services would violate IDEA. School districts therefore cannot establish general rules for deciding which students are eligible for ESY. Each ESY service is determined individually, taking into account the particular circumstances of each student who is potentially in need of such services.

Does ESY apply to students whose third birthdays occur during the summer?

Yes. The US Department of Education has interpreted Part B of IDEA to extend the ESY entitlement to children in preschool programs, including children who reach age 3 during the summer months after being served by Part C (Secs. 300.101[b], 300.323[b]).[1]

SUMMARY

Extended school year services offer students special education and related services beyond the typical school year. ESY services are for students with disabilities who will lose skills or regress during a school break and will have difficulty recouping the skills within a reasonable amount of time after returning to school. As with other decisions about services for students with disabilities, a student's IEP team determines a student's need for ESY services and the types of ESY services to be provided.

REFERENCES

1. 34 CFR Parts 300 (2006).
2. Bar-Lev NB. (1998). Standards for extended school year (ESY). http://www.specialed.us/issues-esy/esymemo.html. Accessed July 10, 2007.
3. *Reusch v Foutain,* 872 F Supp 1421 (D MD 1994).
4. Office of Special Education Programs, US Department of Education. Opinion letter to West Virginia Advocates (February 4, 2003).
5. Gorn S. *What Do I Do When? The Answer Book on Special Education Law*. Horsham, PA: LPR Publications; 1996.

12
The Role of Physical Therapist Assistants In Schools

Sandra Arnold, PT, PhD

A physical therapist assistant (PTA), as described by the American Physical Therapy Association's (APTA) *Guide to Physical Therapist Practice*,[1] is a:

> *... technically educated health care provider who assists the physical therapist in the provision of selected physical therapy interventions. The physical therapist assistant is the only individual who provides selected physical therapy interventions under the direction and supervision of the physical therapist. The physical therapist assistant is a graduate of a physical therapist assistant degree program accredited by the Commission on Accreditation in Physical Therapy Education (CAPTE).*[(p681)]

What is the professional relationship between physical therapists and physical therapist assistants?

APTA describes the physical therapist of record as being directly responsible for the actions of the physical therapist assistant and routinely assesses the ability of the PTA to perform selected and delegated tasks.[1-3] In the document *Utilization of Physical Therapist Assistants in the Provision of Pediatric Physical Therapy*,[4] the APTA Section on Pediatrics recommended that physical therapy services for children who are physiologically unstable not be delegated to the physical therapist assistant. Because credentialing and requirements for utilization of physical therapist assistants vary from state to state, PTs should refer to their state physical therapy practice act and early intervention and special education rules and regulations for additional information specific to their locations.

How does the physical therapist provide "direction and supervision" to the physical therapist assistant?

Direction and supervision of physical therapist assistants are essential for provision of quality physical therapy services.[1-3,5] The type and amount of direction and supervision necessary for assuring quality physical therapy services depend on many factors, including the education and experience of the PTA, the complexity of the child's needs, and the type of intervention planned.[6]

Watts[7] provided a classic guide for physical therapist–physical therapist assistant supervisory relationships. She delineated responsibility through consideration of 5 factors: (1) predictability of the consequences, (2) stability of the situation, (3) observability of basic indicators, (4) ambiguity of basic indicators, and (5) criticality of results. Prior to delegating any physical therapy services, the physical therapist should determine that the consequences of the services are predictable, the situation is stable, and the basic indicators are not ambiguous and do not require ongoing observation and evaluation by the physical therapist. For example, in a home-based early intervention situation in which physical therapy would require ongoing assessment and problem-solving with families, delegation to a physical therapist assistant would not be appropriate.

Supervision of a physical therapist assistant by a physical therapist may vary from direct on-site supervision to general supervision, in which a physical therapist is not routinely on site but is available by telecommunication.[8] The level of supervision will depend upon the responsibilities of the PTA. In addition to the complexity of the child's problems, the type of supervision is "predicated on proximity and accessibility to the physical therapist, supervision available in the event of emergencies or critical events, and type of setting."[6(p2)] In settings where children are likely to experience a change in their status or ability quickly, for example, direct, on-site supervision would be required.

Supervision is directly related to child safety. Verbal and written communication between the physical therapist and the physical therapist assistant and on-site instruction by the physical therapist should be regular and on-going to ensure the child's safety and progress.[5] The physical therapist assistant is responsible for each child's care and safety during service delivery. The PTA should observe and report the child's responses to the supervising physical therapist at regular intervals or in a timely manner if concerns arise.

The PTA and supervising PT should work with administrators at the local and state levels to ensure that their professional roles and responsibilities are clearly defined. The person who directs physical therapy services in an early intervention program, school, or district should: (1) establish guidelines that describe the role and responsibilities of the PTA in the services and the supervisory relationships inherent in the environment; (2) ensure that physical therapy services are provided efficiently and effectively and in accordance with safe and legal physical therapy practice; (3) interpret administrative policies; (4) act as a liaison between the PTA and administration, if necessary; and (5) foster the professional growth of the PTA.[1,6]

Note that the supervising physical therapist must be properly credentialed in the jurisdiction in which the physical therapist assistant is delivering services. This can be a concern if a physical therapist supervises a physical therapist assistant in another state.

What is the role of a PTA in a school setting?

Generally, in the school setting, the physical therapist assistant is professionally responsible to and under the supervision and direction of a licensed physical therapist for all delivery of service-related functions. The PTA is considered a team member and may provide input, along with the physical therapist, when establishing educational goals for a student that will be documented in the student's individualized education program (IEP). After the IEP team develops the student's goals, the team determines whether or not physical therapy services will assist the student to benefit from the educational program. If physical therapy will enable the student to benefit from special education, the team, with input from the physical therapist, will define the frequency and duration of the services needed. The PT may delegate aspects of the student's physical therapy to a PTA that are appropriate for the student's needs and the PTA's experience, knowledge, and skill. (For more information, see the question related to appropriate roles for PTAs in classrooms and other natural settings in this chapter.) The physical therapist will design a plan to meet the IEP goals, and the PTA may follow through and assist with the physical therapy plan as delegated and directed by the physical therapist. A PTA may modify specific interventions established by the physical therapist in response to change in a student's status, but may not change the plan of care.[5] If on a particular day a student complains of being tired, for example, a PTA could decrease a planned activity or exercise for that particular day.

The APTA Section on Pediatrics document "Utilization of Physical Therapist Assistants in Various Pediatric Setting"[9] provides 2 examples of the roles of PTA in public school settings. In the Sumner School District in Washington State, responsibilities of the physical therapist assistant include:

- Implements and documents therapy programs and may assist students with special equipment including positioning, exercise, developmental motor programs, ambulation, and functional lifetime activities

- Assists the physical therapist in complex procedures and evaluations
- Assists the physical therapist in gathering, organizing, and reporting assessment data
- Manages equipment, schedule, workplace, and therapy files
- Other duties assigned and needed for efficient functioning within the classroom.[9]

The North Carolina Department of Public Instruction Division of Exceptional Children's Services described the major functions of the PTA as:

- Identification—The physical therapist assistant assists the physical therapist in observing and screening students with physical/motor disabilities.
- Program management—The physical therapist assistant participates in the local education agency's comprehensive planning process for the education of exceptional children and assists the physical therapist in the management and maintenance of the physical therapy program.
- Education—The physical therapist assistant assists the physical therapist providing information to establish relationships with school personnel, parents, and non-school agencies to facilitate the education of students with physical/motor disabilities.[9]

Can a PTA perform administrative and/or screening activities?

Yes. A physical therapist assistant may follow established administrative procedures, including keeping records and inventory, ordering supplies and equipment, and scheduling, in consultation with the supervising therapist. The physical therapist may ask the physical therapist assistant, if appropriately trained and knowledgeable and as permissible by state practice act/laws, to assist in screenings (such as for scoliosis), participate in school-wide education, perform selected measurement procedures, and care for braces, orthoses, prostheses, and adaptive equipment.[10] The PT should consider the PTA's experience, participation in continuing education courses, and education in other areas, such as psychology, early childhood development, or special education when delegating duties such as screening and measurement procedures.[4]

If supervised, can a PTA perform all school-based physical therapy services?

No. A school-based physical therapist assistant should not interpret any student referrals, evaluate or reevaluate students, determine physical therapy diagnosis or prognosis, develop or modify a student's physical therapy plan (educational program), determine utilization of the PTA, release or discharge a student from physical therapy services, recommend wheelchairs, orthoses, prostheses, or other assistive devices, or alterations to architectural barriers to persons other than a physical therapist, or perform any skills or activities that are beyond the knowledge base of the physical therapist assistant.[1,3,6] A PTA delivers only those interventions selected by the PT and within the knowledge base of the PTA (eg, the PTA has the responsibility *not* to perform a certain service if not qualified, even if the PT delegates it).[5]

Must a physical therapist document activities of a PTA?

Requirements for documentation vary from state to state and from program to program.[11] If a physical therapist has delegated a plan of care to be implemented by a PTA, the physical therapist must document the delegation of activities and services the PTA will provide.[4] The physical therapist also is responsible for the oversight of all documentation for services provided for the child.[6]

Are PTAs required to be licensed?

State law, primarily through licensure in most United States jurisdictions, regulates physical therapist assistants.[12] Physical therapist assistant members of the American Physical Therapy Association are also bound by the *APTA Standards of Ethical Conduct for the Physical Therapist Assistant* and the *Guide for Conduct of the Physical Therapist Assistant*.[3,5]

Is a physical therapist responsible for services provided by a PTA?

Yes. The supervising physical therapist is ultimately responsible for the provision of all physical therapy services.[6] A PTA should provide services in a manner that is consistent with safe, legal, and ethical physical therapy practice.[3, 5] The PT should be cognizant of the PTA's education and scope of knowledge and should ensure that the PTA follows state regulatory mandates and ethical professional standards.

How are physical therapy aides utilized in an early intervention or school setting?

APTA defines physical therapy aides as non-licensed workers who are specifically trained under the direction of a physical therapist.[1] Physical therapy aides provide support that may include child-related and non-child-related duties only with continuous on-site supervision by the physical therapist or by the PTA where allowed by law or regulation.[1]

How does the IEP team decide if other assistants or paraprofessionals can carry certain tasks?

This is not an easy question to answer. Direction for the use of other assistants and paraprofessionals is being established by individual states to address current concerns about: (1) a critical shortage of personnel to meet service demand, (2) specialized training required to provide services to young children, (3) distance and travel time constraints, (4) fully inclusive placement for children and students, and (5) budget and monetary constraints.[13] States and other jurisdictions are guided by their own unique needs as they address appropriate roles of personnel providing services for students with disabilities.

Unfortunately, establishing guidelines around these concerns may not be in the best interest of children, families, or professionals. The team is responsible for selecting the most appropriate person to provide each service. The "most appropriate" individual on the team is the person who is best qualified and has the knowledge base and experiences needed within the particular area of service. As an example, an IEP team might agree that a student's goal is to use the restroom independently and that physical therapy services are needed to assist the student to learn to transfer from the wheelchair to the toilet seat. The team, with input from the physical therapist, would determine which team member is the most appropriate to provide transfer training. If the student was new to the district and had not previously attempted toilet transfers, the physical therapist might initially be responsible for the physical therapy services. Later, after determining how best to teach the student to transfer, the PT might delegate the service delivery to the physical therapist assistant. If, however, the student is well-known to the physical therapist and only needs continued practice, the most appropriate team member to begin intervention might be the physical therapist assistant. If the student is proficient in toilet transfers but just needs help unsnapping pants, for example, then the paraprofessional in the classroom might be the only person needed for the student to carry out the activity.

What are appropriate roles for PTAs in classrooms and other natural settings that are not appropriate for teachers and classroom paraprofessionals?

Teachers and paraprofessionals also may assist students with motor-related activities that are within the scope of their education and experience, that they can carry out safely, and that can be provided in accordance with applicable laws and regulations.[1] When physical therapists make recommendations to classroom staff for positioning, promoting motor function, or similar activities, they are responsible for ensuring that the staff have the necessary skills and knowledge. Physical therapist assistants should not make such recommendations. Physical therapist assistants may modify an intervention within the scope of the physical therapy plan of care according to changes in student status, but teachers or paraprofessionals should not modify a specific approach.[1,5] If a teacher or paraprofessional observed that a student was leaning to the right in a wheelchair, for example, it would not be appropriate to alter the wheelchair without first receiving an assessment and recommendation from the PT. The PTA may provide students/families with information about provision of physical therapy services, such as how and when the services will be delivered, the expected progression, and the expected outcomes; however, a teacher or paraprofessional should not.[1,5] Physical therapist assistants implement the IEP plan of care and can instruct parents, teachers, and paraprofessionals in specific strategies, such as positioning or transfers.

Are appropriate roles for aides and assistants becoming any clearer?

In the area of early intervention and preschool services, individual states are defining appropriate roles of personnel through the development of: (1) policy and personnel standards, (2) new occupational categories at the paraprofessional level, (3) personnel standards, and (4) credentialing processes.[13] A 1995 survey of chief state school officers conducted by the National Resource Center for Paraprofessionals in Education and Related Services reported, however, that less than half (24) of the states had established guidelines for paraprofessional roles, duties, supervision, and training at that time.[15] Maryland has established a credentialing system for paraeducators, and Utah has approved standards for the employment, training, and supervision of paraprofessionals employed in special education. The Idaho Division of Vocational Education, with the assistance of a committee representing different education and related services providers and higher education personnel from preparation programs, has developed task lists and curriculum guides for aides and assistants who support speech-language pathologists and physical and occupational therapists.[14] In an attempt to ensure the availability of appropriately trained personnel, states and other jurisdictions will continue to integrate assistants and paraprofessionals into their systems. State physical therapy associations and individual physical therapists should be involved with the policy decision making in their states.

SUMMARY

Physical therapist assistants may serve as members of teams and assist physical therapists in the provision of physical therapy services. They may provide services under the direction and supervision of an appropriately licensed physical therapist and should follow professional standards of practice and ethical conduct. Physical therapist assistants' roles will vary according to program policies and the practice acts of the states in which they work.

REFERENCES

1. *Guide to Physical Therapist Practice. Revised* 2nd ed. Alexandria, VA: American Physical Therapy Association; 2003.
2. APTA Guide for Professional Conduct. Alexandria, VA: American Physical Therapy Association; 2004. http://www.apta.org/AM/Template.cfm?Section=Core_Documents1&Template=/CM/HTMLDisplay.cfm&ContentID=24781. Accessed July 10, 2007.
3. APTA Standards of Ethical Conduct for the Physical Therapist Assistant (HOD 06-00-13-24). House of Delegates policy. American Physical Therapy Association Web site. http://www.apta.org/AM/Template.cfm?Section=Scope_of_Work_Supervision1&Template=/CM/HTMLDisplay.cfm&ContentID=23729. Accessed July 10, 2007.
4. *Utilization of the Physical Therapist Assistants in the Provision of Pediatric Physical Therapy.* Alexandria, VA: American Physical Therapy Association; 1997.
5. Guide for Conduct of the Physical Therapist Assistant. Alexandria, VA: American Physical Therapy Association; 2004. http://www.apta.org/AM/Template.cfm?Section=Scope_of_Work_Supervision1&Template=/CM/HTMLDisplay.cfm&ContentID=23731. Accessed July 10, 2007.
6. Direction and Supervision of the Physical Therapist Assistant (HOD P06-05-18-26). House of Delegates policy. American Physical Therapy Association Web site. http://www.apta.org/AM/Template.cfm?Section=Policies_and_Bylaws&TEMPLATE=/CM/ContentDisplay.cfm&CONTENTID=25672. Accessed July 10, 2007.
7. Watts NT. Task analysis and division of responsibility in physical therapy. *Phys Ther.* 1971;51:23-35.
8. Levels of Supervision (HOD P06-00-15-26). House of Delegates policy. American Physical Therapy Association Web site. http://www.apta.org/AM/Template.cfm?Section=Policies_and_Bylaws&TEMPLATE=/CM/ContentDisplay.cfm&CONTENTID=25508. Accessed July 10, 2007.
9. *Utilization of Physical Therapist Assistants in Various Pediatric Settings.* Alexandria, VA: American Physical Therapy Association, Section on Pediatrics; 1996.
10. Martin KD, ed. *Physical Therapy Practice in Educational Environments: Policies and Guidelines.* Alexandria, VA: American Physical Therapy Association Section on Pediatrics; 1990.
11. Guidelines: Physical Therapy Documentation of Patient/Client Management (HOD G03-05-16-41). House of Delegates policy. American Physical Therapy Association Web site. http://www.apta.org/AM/Template.cfm?Section=Policies_and_Bylaws&TEMPLATE=/CM/ContentDisplay.cfm&CONTENTID=31688. Accessed July 10, 2007.
12. Physical Therapist and Physical Therapist Assistant Licensure/Regulation (HOD P05-07-09-10). House of Delegates policy. American Physical Therapy Association Web site. http://www.apta.org/AM/Template.cfm?Section=Policies_and_Bylaws&TEMPLATE=/CM/ContentDisplay.cfm&CONTENTID=25398. Accessed July 10, 2007.

13. Striffler N. *Current Trends in the Use of Paraprofessionals in Early Intervention and Preschool Services.* Chapel Hill, NC: National Early Childhood Technical Assistance System; 1993.
14. Picket A. *A State of the Art Report on Paraeducators in Education and Related Services.* New York, NY: The Graduate School and University Center, City University of New York; 1996.

13
Third-Party Payment for Physical Therapy Under IDEA

Maria Jones, PT, PhD, ATP, and Amanda Porter, PT, MPT

As the number of children receiving special education and related services increases, local education agencies continue to look for additional funding sources to pay for the services provided in the educational environment. Sec. 300.103 says:

> *Each State may use whatever State, local, Federal, and private sources of support are available in the State to meet the requirements of (Part B)... Nothing in this part relieves an insurer or similar third party from an otherwise valid obligation to provide or pay for services provided to a child (with a disability)... the State must ensure that there is no delay in implementing a child's IEP, including any case in which the payment source for providing or paying for special education and related services to the child is being determined.*

Does this mean that schools can bill Medicaid for physical therapy?

Yes. Sec. 300.154(d)(1) states, "A public agency may use the Medicaid or other public benefits or insurance programs in which a child participates to provide or pay for services required under this part (Part B), as permitted under the public benefits or insurance program." Therefore, school districts can bill for physical therapy and other related services provided in the educational environment.[1-4] Congress anticipated that local school districts would use Medicaid and other resources available under other federal laws for the education of students with disabilities served under IDEA.[4] The Centers for Medicare and Medicaid Services (CMS) have determined that school districts can bill for health-related services provided for students enrolled in Medicaid; however, the services must be medically necessary.

What is the Medicaid definition of "medically necessary?"

Because Medicaid is a state-administered medical assistance program, each state develops its own definitions and guidelines regarding eligibility and services.[4] No standard definition of medical necessity exists. Although some states require physical therapists to obtain a physician's referral for a service to be considered medically necessary, other states do not have such a requirement. PTs should contact the agency that manages the state's Medicaid program for the specific definition of medical necessity, including the requirement for physician's referral and documentation.

Can services be both medically necessary and educationally relevant?

Yes. In the case of Massachusetts v Secretary of HHS,[5] the First Circuit Court of Appeals determined that a violation of the Medicaid law occurred when a blanket exclusion of special education services was made and reimbursement for these services was denied.[6] The court ruled that the concepts represented by "education" and "medical assistance" overlap and that investigation into "the nature of the services, not just into what they are called or who provides them, must be made to determine appropriate billing options."[5] With parental consent, school districts can seek reimbursement for physical therapy services from public or private insurance companies even though they are provided in the educational environment.

Can a school require parents to enroll in Medicaid for their children to receive physical therapy as a related service?

No. Sec. 300.154(d)(2)(i) says, "the public agency may not require parents to sign up for or enroll in public benefits or insurance programs in order for their child to receive FAPE...." Schools may not use Medicaid eligibility to determine if a child requires physical therapy services to receive a FAPE. Once an IEP team determines that a child requires physical therapy, the team can ask if a student is enrolled in Medicaid and, with parental consent, may seek reimbursement for those services.

Can a school district bill a family's insurance company for school-based physical therapy?

Sec. 300.103(a) says school districts "may use whatever State, local, federal, and private sources of support are available in the State to meet the requirements of this part." Sec. 300.103(b) further says that "nothing in this part relieves an insurer or similar third party for an otherwise valid obligation to provide or pay for services provided to a child with a disability." Sec. 300.154(e)(1), however, says that school districts may access a parent's private insurance only if the parents provide informed consent to the school district. More specifically, Sec. 300.154(e)(2)(i-ii) says that school districts must obtain parental consent every time they access the parent's private insurance and must inform parents that refusal to permit the school district to access their private insurance does not relieve the school districts of its responsibility to provide all necessary services at no cost to the parent.[7]

What does "at no cost to the parent" mean?

If school districts bill for physical therapy or other services, they must ensure that parents do not incur costs either currently or in the future. Sec. 300.154(d)(2)(ii) states "school districts cannot require parents to incur an out-of-pocket expense such as payment of a deductible or co-pay amount incurred in filing a claim for services." School districts can, however, pay the cost that the parents would be required to pay, including such deductibles and co-pays. Sec. 300.154(d)(2)(iii) specifies that school districts cannot use public or private insurance to pay for services if such use would:

- (A) *decrease in available lifetime coverage or any other insured benefit;*
- (B) *result in the family paying for services that would otherwise be covered by the public benefits or insurance program and that are required for the child outside of the time the child is in school;*
- (C) *increase premiums or lead to the discontinuation of benefits or insurance; or*
- (D) *risk loss of eligibility for home and community-based waivers, based on aggregate health-related expenditures.*[3,4]

If a school requests Medicaid or private insurance information, do parents have to provide it?

No. Parents are not required to provide the school with this information. If parents choose to provide such information, school districts must still obtain parental consent prior to billing any third party for services provided as part of the student's educational program. Schools cannot make provision of physical therapy or other special education or related services contingent on a parent's consent to bill a third party. Parents may refuse to consent without jeopardizing their child's rights to special education and related services determined by the IEP team to be necessary to meet the child's unique needs.[8]

If a parent provides consent to bill for services provided in the educational environment, but has to pay a deductible each year, can the school district pay the family's deductible?

Yes. The school district can use Part B funds to prevent the family from incurring costs such as deductibles or copayments. Sec. 300.154(f)(2) states:

> *... to avoid financial cost to parents who otherwise would consent to use private insurance, or public insurance if the parent would incur a cost, the public agency may use its Part B funds to pay the cost the parents otherwise would have to pay to use the parent's benefits or insurance (e.g., the deductible or co-pay amounts).*

Can a school district delay physical therapy until they get approval from Medicaid and/or private insurance?

No. The school district must implement physical therapy in a timely manner, once the team has determined such services are needed and included them on the child's IEP. Sec. 300.103(c) says:

> *... the State must ensure that there is no delay in implementing a child's IEP, including any case in which the payment source for providing or paying for special education and related services to the child is being determined.*

Billing Medicaid and/or private insurance typically requires the use of CPT® codes. What are CPT codes?

Current Procedural Terminology (CPT®) codes are used for reporting the medical services and procedures provided to an individual. The codes are intended to provide common terminology, allowing medical services providers, patients, and insurers to communicate. CPT codes are updated annually.[9]

How are CPT codes used and how do physical therapists determine which codes to use?

Physical therapists use CPT codes to file claims or bill for the services they provide. The definitions of various CPT codes are listed in the annually published CPT coding manual[9] and physical therapists should read them to determine which codes most accurately describe the services they provide for children in early intervention or students in the educational environment. Some examples of CPT codes and their descriptors that might be appropriate for services provided under IDEA Parts C and B[9]:

97110	*Therapeutic procedure, one or more areas, each 15 minutes; therapeutic exercises to develop strength and endurance, range of motion and flexibility* (p428)
97112	*Therapeutic procedure, one or more areas, each 15 minutes; neuromuscular reeducation of movement, balance, coordination, kinesthetic sense, posture, and/or proprioception for sitting and/or standing activities* (p428)
97116	*Therapeutic procedure, one or more areas, each 15 minutes; gait training (includes stair climbing)* (p428)
97530	*Therapeutic activities, direct (one-on-one) patient contact by the provider (use of dynamic activities to improve functional performance), each 15 minutes* (p429)
97535	*Self-care/home management training (eg, activities of daily living (ADL) and compensatory training, meal preparation, safety procedures, and instructions in use of assistive technology devices/adaptive equipment) direct one-on-one contact by provider, each 15 minutes* (p429)
97537	*Community/work reintegration training (eg, shopping, transportation, money management, avocational activities and/or work environment/modification analysis, work task analysis, use of assistive technology device/adaptive equipment), direct one-on-one contact by provider, each 15 minutes* (p429)
97542	*Wheelchair management (eg, assessment, fitting, training), each 15 minutes* (p429)
97755	*Assistive technology assessment (eg, to restore, augment or compensate for existing function, optimize functional tasks and/or maximize environmental accessibility), direct one-on-one contact by provider, with written report, each 15 minutes* (p430)

For more information and more codes, refer to the CPT coding manual.[9]

SUMMARY

Early intervention programs and school districts, with parental consent, may bill third-party payers for physical therapy and other services. Medicaid is the most common payer, but programs also may bill other third-party payers, as long as parents will not incur current or future costs.

REFERENCES

1. Bohmert J, David K, Glickman L, Wallis K. Task force report on third party reimbursement in the school. *Pediatr Phys Ther.* 1990;2:114-116.
2. Weber MC. The legal and policy implications of third party reimbursement for early childhood services. *J Early Interv.* 1991;15(3):298-303.
3. Rogers JJ. *Third Party Billing for Special Education: Panacea or Mirage?* Cambridge, MA: Brookline Books; 1993.
4. Lewin/ICF and Fox Health Policy Consultants. *Medicaid Coverage of Health-Related Services for Children Receiving Special Education: An Examination of Federal Policies.* Washington, DC: US Government Printing Office; 1991. ERIC Document Reproduction Service ED347753..
5. *Massachusetts v Secretary of HHS,* 816 F2d 796 (1st Cir 1987).
6. U.S. Department of Health and Human Services. *Medicaid Coverage of Health-Related Services for Children Receiving Special Education: An Examination of Federal Policies.* Washington, DC: Government Printing Office; 1991.
7. Schrag JA. Letter to Spann, 20 Individuals With Disabilities Education Law Report (IDELR) 627 (1993).
8. Davila RR. Letter to Simon, 17 Education for the Handicapped Law Reporter (EHLR) 225 (1990).
9. American Medical Association. *Physicians' Current Procedural Terminology.* Professional ed. Chicago, IL: American Medical Association; 2007.

14 Transportation

Maria Jones, PT, PhD, ATP, and Amanda Porter, PT, MPT

Transportation is one of the many related services that school districts must provide for student with disabilities who need it. Specifically, Sec. 300.34(16)(i-iii) says:

> *Transportation includes travel to and from school and between schools; travel in and around school buildings; and specialized equipment (such as special or adapted buses, lifts, and ramps), if required to provide special transportation for a child with a disability.*

Sec. 300.107 also includes transportation as a nonacademic and extracurricular service that may be necessary to provide "*an equal opportunity for participation in those services and activities.*" The regulations, however, provide little guidance for a school district's transportation responsibilities and requirements. Physical therapists, who are often involved in assisting children with mobility, can play an important role in determining specific transportation needs.

How does a district determine if a student requires transportation?

Decisions about transportation are made through the IEP process. The Office of Special Education Programs (OSEP) said:

> *… each student's need for transportation as a related service and the type of transportation to be provided are issues to be discussed and decided during the evaluation process and individualized education program (IEP) meeting, and the transportation arrangements agreed upon should be included in the disabled student's IEP.*[1]

Are bus drivers considered members of the IEP team?

If an IEP team decides a student requires specialized transportation as a related service, transportation staff should be invited to participate in development of the IEP. The transportation staff need information about the student's unique needs related to safety, which other IEP team member can provide. In turn, the transportation staff can provide such information as the type and configuration of the vehicle, probable length of ride, pickup/drop-off procedures, type of device and occupant securement system, degree of training and skills of the driver, and need for a bus attendant.[1]

Are school districts required to provide door-to-door transportation for all students with disabilities?

No. Neither IDEA[2] nor Section 504 of the Rehabilitation Act[3] define a district's responsibility for the exact locations where a student is picked-up and dropped off. OSEP advises districts to make such decisions as part of the IEP and on a case-by-case basis.[4] As a general rule, districts should consider "the student's age, the nature of the student's disability, the student's ability to move independently, the distance between home and the bus stop, the nature and conditions of the route to and from the bus stop and the availability of, and access to, public assistance"[5] when deciding between bus stop assignment and door-to-door transportation.

Can schools require a parent to provide transportation?

If a student requires transportation as a related service, the school district must provide it at no cost to the parent.[1] Even if the district does not offer transportation to students in general education, the district has an obligation under IDEA to provide transportation for students in special education who require it. If, however, students with disabilities can use the same transportation services as students in general education, transportation does not have to be listed as a related service on the IEP.[6]

Can parents request reimbursement for transportation they provide?

Yes. OSEP has clarified, however, that IDEA does not address whether parents are entitled to reimbursement for transporting their child to school when transportation is listed as a required related service in the IEP.[1] School districts frequently provide reimbursement of mileage costs to a parent or relative providing transportation or pay for public or private transportation when deemed necessary.

What training should bus drivers and other transportation staff receive?

Because bus drivers and attendants will have responsibility for the student and specialized equipment during transportation, they should receive training to understand how to: (1) use proper body mechanics and lifting techniques, (2) operate equipment, (3) appropriately secure students (occupants) and equipment, and (4) manage student behavior. OSEP supports transportation staff being informed and trained.[7]

How should wheelchairs and students be secured during transport?

The 1994 amendments to the federal Motor Vehicle Safety Standards and Regulations (FMVSS) 222 (School Bus Passenger Seating and Crash Protection)[7] established safety requirements for securing wheelchairs and wheelchair occupants on school buses. Whenever possible or feasible, students should be transferred out of wheelchairs and positioned in a regular bus or car seat that meets safety standards.

To determine whether transfers are feasible, the team should consider how much assistance the student needs to transfer and if the student can maintain an upright sitting posture without wheelchair supports. If transferring students is not feasible, safe transportation requires use of four-point wheelchair securement straps, which anchor the wheelchair to the bus/vehicle, and separate occupant restraints to secure the student to the wheelchair. Occupant restraints are not part of the student's wheelchair, but are three-point harnesses that attach to the frame of the bus and are positioned around the student during transportation, much like a traditional seatbelt in a car.[8-9]

Some wheelchairs are designed as transit models and have specific attachment points for wheelchair securement straps. Other wheelchairs do not have such attachment points, but can still be safely transported. For wheelchairs that do not have specific attachment points, the wheelchair securement straps should be anchored to the frame of the chair, not a moving part of the chair, such as the wheels, armrest, or footrests.[8-9]

Students often have seat belts and shoulder/chest straps on their wheelchairs. Can such straps be used instead of occupant restraints?

No. The use of postural supports, such as seat belts and shoulder straps, are intended to support the student in upright alignment and are often essential for the occupant restraint system to work effectively; however, they are not designed as occupant restraints, are not crash-tested, and should never be used alone. If problems with the student's postural alignment are observed, the team should consult with a physical therapist to determine possible solutions to the identified problems.[8-9]

Are the brakes on a student's wheelchair sufficient for securing the chair during transport?

No. Brakes alone are not sufficient for securing a student's chair during transport and are not considered a component of the wheelchair securement system. Brakes, however, should be used to stabilize the wheelchair when using a bus lift.

When should car seats and seat belts be used?

When a student can transfer to the vehicle seat and use the original equipment manufacturer occupant restraints (eg, seat/lap belts), then such restraints should be used. Young children or any child weighing less than 50 pounds should be secured in an appropriate child restraint or safety vest meeting the requirements of FMVSS 213.[10]

If students have trays, communication devices, and other equipment, should they remain on the student's wheelchair?

No. Wheelchair trays, communication devices, and any other equipment should be removed during transit and stored/secured to avoid them from becoming projectiles in the event of an accident.[8-9]

Are students transported in wheelchairs required to have headrests?

Individual state and district policies vary; however, IEP teams should consider the student's need for a headrest during transit, just as they would in an automobile. As a general rule, students should have a headrest or proper head/neck support to avoid whiplash injuries in the event of an accident. The student's head should not be restrained to a headrest with straps or any other external devices. If a student's wheelchair does not have a headrest, the IEP team may want to consider having the student transfer to a seat that provides a headrest. IEP teams must understand, however, that wheelchair headrests are often not crash-tested and may not prevent injury in the event of an accident.[11]

If a student is transported in a wheelchair, which direction should the chair/student face?

Students who are transported in a wheelchair should face the front of the bus.[8]

SUMMARY

Transportation can be an important service that districts must provide for students with disabilities who require it. Although IDEA provides little guidance concerning specific transportation requirements, local school districts have to ensure compliance with IDEA,[2] as well as Section 504 of the Rehabilitation Act of 1975,[3] the Americans with Disabilities Act,[12] and the federal Motor Vehicle Safety Standards and Regulations.[5] IEP team members should work together to clearly define students' specific transportation needs, provide appropriate training to all staff responsible for transportation, and monitor compliance with local and state policies and procedures.

REFERENCES

1. Lee SS. Letter to Anonymous, 38 Individuals With Disabilities Education Law Report (IDELR) 42 (2002).
2. Public Law 108-446, Individuals With Disabilities Education Improvement Act of 2004. Available at http://www.copyright.gov/legislation/pl108-446.pdf. Accessed December 12, 2007.
3. Public Law 93-112, Rehabilitation Act (1973), 29 USC§794.
4. Hehir T. Letter to Smith, 23 Individuals With Disabilities Education Law Report (IDELR) 344 (1995).
5. Lake SE. *Transporting Students with Disabilities: A Legal Overview.* Horsham, Pa: LRP Publications; 2005.
6. Hehir T. Letter to Hamilton, 25 Individuals With Disabilities Education Law Report (IDELR) 520 (1996).
7. Lee SS. Memorandum to State Directors of Education, 40 Individuals With Disabilities Education Law Report (IDELR) 155 (2003).
8. National Highway Traffic Safety Administration Web site. *Safety Standards.* http://www.nhtsa.dot.gov/cars/rules/standards/. Accessed June 22, 2007.
9. American Academy of Pediatrics Committee on Injury and Poison Prevention. School bus transportation of children with special health care needs. *Pediatr.* 2001;102:516-518.
10. National Highway Traffic Safety Administration. *Guideline for the Safe Transportation of Pre-school Age Children in School Buses.* Washington, DC: National Highway Traffic Safety Administration; 1999.
11. Karg P, Sprigle S. Development of test methodologies for determining the safety of wheelchair headrest systems during vehicle transport. *J Rehabil Res Develop. 1996;33(3):290-304.*
12. Public Law 101-336, Americans With Disabilities Act (1990), 42 USC§12101.

Section II:
Due Process Decisions

Court Decisions, State Education Agency Hearings, Letters of Inquiry, Policy Interpretation, and Investigations by Federal Agencies Related to School-Based Physical Therapy

Maria Jones, PT, PhD, ATP, and Mary Jane Rapport, PT, PhD

Although physical therapy may be included as a related service that students with disabilities receive as part of their individualized education programs (IEP), parents and school personnel do not always agree with all aspects of the plan, including how, when, where, and what physical therapy services should be provided. When disagreements occur, parents may seek to resolve a dispute with a school district by using due process procedures, as described in Chapter 2. School-based physical therapy services have been the focal point of a variety of due process or court decisions.

Children receiving special education and related services under IDEA have an IEP based on their unique needs. Although the decision-making process used to resolve disputes may be similar for all children, the outcomes of due process decisions are influenced by the individual needs of the child and the child's educational situation. When reviewing past legal decisions, therefore, caution must be taken to avoid assuming that a new dispute will yield the same outcome as a similar situation preceding it. Many of the past disagreements leading to due process hearings have involved: (1) adequacy of physical therapy services; (2) qualification and training of personnel; (3) need for physical therapy during the summer or extended school breaks; (4) compensatory physical therapy services; and (5) type of intervention provided as physical therapy. Other disagreements, including access to third-party reimbursement, method of service delivery, and independent physical therapy evaluations, also have been addressed, although less frequently. The process and timelines for how parents and school districts should proceed when disagreements occur are described in Sec. 300.508.

This chapter provides an overview of due process decisions at state and federal levels. Resolutions reached through mediation or following an initial due process hearing at the local education agency level are not included because this information is not available through public sources. The disagreements addressed in this chapter have been appealed to decision makers at multiple levels of due process from the state education agency to state and federal courts. The chapter also summarizes letters of interpretation by the US Department of Education and findings of the Office of Civil Rights. These documents from the federal agencies that oversee access to education and the rights of children with disabilities provide clarification from key components in the regulatory and compliance processes.

Knowing which decisions and interpretations are persuasive in a particular state or local education agency and which are mandatory or controlling is important. Understanding this requires a brief overview of the US judicial organizational structure. The US Supreme Court is the highest judicial body, and it decides cases and provides opinions that become mandatory across all jurisdictions in the country. The next highest judicial level is the US federal Circuit Courts of Appeals and just below that are more than 90 US District Courts. A decision in a federal district court sets precedence in the entire jurisdiction, or geographical area, covered by that particular court. If a disagreement occurs in another region, outside the federal district court that rendered the previous decision, the original decision would be persuasive and could be used to guide other parties located outside the controlling jurisdiction. Only a decision from within the same federal jurisdiction, or from a higher court with broader authority, however, would be considered as more than guidance or persuasive opinion. An opinion set by a hearing officer or state education agency (SEA) in one state, for example, is mandatory over all school districts in that same state, but is only persuasive or guiding for a similar situation in another state.

Opinions that have persuasive authority may be influential or convincing in future decisions when disagreements are similar to the original, and their relevance should not be disregarded in other parts of the country. Careful review of all cases and decisions involving the delivery of physical therapy as a related service whether or not the situation is identical or has occurred in a school district nearby or within the same state is important. Tables 1-6 provide summaries of federal and state judicial decisions, state education agency hearings, and letters of inquiry, policy interpretation, and investigations by federal agencies to complaints or inquiries with formal requests for clarification; all related to provision of physical therapy under IDEA. Decisions related to assistive technology are included in Chapter 10.

The tables are organized by jurisdiction, or level of authority, and then entries are listed in chronological order (starting with the most recent) within each level or section. The tables provide only a summary, so physical therapists should locate and read decisions in their entirety before applying them to a new scenario or situation. Citations to the IDELR (Individuals With Disabilities Education Law Report),[1] formerly the EHLR (Education of the Handicapped Law Report),[2] refer to a loose-leaf publication from the LRP Publishing Company. All of the documents referenced in the tables are public information and can be obtained through multiple avenues via the Internet or as hard copies. Assistance in locating the documents can be obtained in many state departments of education, special education regional resource centers, larger university education or law libraries, and law firms specializing in education law.

The tables include all items from the first edition of this book and also includes the more recent decisions since the original publication. Relatively few changes occurred in the types of cases that have come before hearing officers and judges in the courts during these past 8 years. Overall, the legal disparities primarily focus on adequacy of the physical therapy services provided by the school district, frequency of physical therapy services, and requests for compensatory physical therapy services when services have not been provided or not adequately provided as specified in the IEP. Disagreements continue between parents and school districts on the extent to which a student needs physical therapy or the extent to which existing personnel will fulfill the district's obligations as outlined in the IEP. Occasional disagreements occur on the type of intervention or method of service delivery, but resolutions for such disagreements are not sought frequently. The need for compensatory services, or the request to provide services to "make up" for "missed" physical therapy would not exist if *each* school district fulfilled *each* IEP as agreed upon by the parent and the school district during development of the student's educational program.

When reviewing the tables, focus on the decisions that are controlling in your state and the issues addressed by the same state education agency or decided in the same federal court jurisdiction. Reviewing decisions that may be persuasive because they appear to focus on a very similar situation or scenario also is helpful. The letters of clarification by the US Department of Education provide general clarification that often goes beyond the federal regulations or simplifies an issue. The letters of finding from the other federal agencies are also relevant because they provide guidance on similar issues that school districts have had to address. Above all, each entry sheds light on the types of disagreements that continue to confront school districts and parents as all parties work to provide a program that will assist students to benefit from their education and reach satisfactory levels of independence.

REFERENCES

1. Individuals With Disabilities Education Law Report. West Palm Beach, FL: LRP Publications.
2. Education of the Handicapped Law Report. West Palm Beach, FL: LRP Publications.

Table 1. Court Decisions, Letters of Inquiry, and Policy Interpretation Related to School-Based Physical Therapy: US Supreme Court Decisions

Case	Citation	Jurisdiction/Year	Issue	Comments
Cedar Rapids Community Sch. Dist. v Garret F	29 IDELR 966, S.Ct.	S.Ct. 1999	Provision of related services	Provision of continuous nursing service was a related service that the district was required to provide under IDEA because it was a supportive service and was not an excluded medical service.
Irving Independent School District v Tatro	468 U.S. 833, 104 S.Ct. 3371	S.Ct. 1984	Provision of related services	Provision of intermittent catheterization was a related service under the Education of the Handicapped Act (EHA) and not a medical service. Attorney fees were available under the Act and awarded to the parents. This case established the "bright-line test," defining that "the services of a physician (other than for diagnostic and evaluation purposes) are subject to the medical services exclusion, but services that can be provided in the school setting by a nurse or qualified layperson are not."

Table 2. Court Decisions, Letters of Inquiry, and Policy Interpretation Related to School-Based Physical Therapy: Federal Court of Appeals Decisions

Case	Citation	Jurisdiction/Year	Issue	Comments
Peck by Peck v Lansing Sch. Dist.	28 IDELR 472	6th Cir. 1998	Location of physical therapy services	The court determined that the school could provide physical therapy services on the premises of a parochial school "without excessive entanglement of government and religion in violation of the Establishment Clause of the U.S. Constitution."
Chester County Intermediate Unit v Pennsylvania Blue Shield	896 F.2d 808	3rd Cir. 1990	Third-party reimbursement	Court determined that EHA made clear that only government is financially responsible for related services such as physical therapy. Court further held that parents were not entitled to relief from private health insurers because policies only covered reimbursements to subscribers who paid deductible on claims for charges they actually incurred.
Polk v Central Susquehanna Intermediate Unit No. 16	853 F.2d 171	3rd Cir. 1988	Service provider	School district policy of refusing to consider direct PT by a licensed therapist could not be resolved; however, the case was remanded to district court for further consideration of this issue. This case also examined the provision of PT using a consultative model of service delivery and the need to provide "some educational benefit" (Rowley standard) that was more than de minimus, or trivial.

The following abbreviations are included in Tables 1-6:

ADHD = Attention deficit hyperactivity disorder
Bd = Board
CP = Cerebral palsy
Cir. = Circuit; refers to federal appellate court
Dist = District
Educ = Education
EHA = Education of Handicapped Act
EHLR = Education of Handicapped Law Report
EHLR DEC. = Education of Handicapped Law Report Decision: citation used to locate a judicial decision in the EHLR
ESY = Extended school year
FAPE = Free and appropriate public education
IDEA = Individuals with Disabilities Education Act
IDELR = Individuals with Disabilities Education Law Report: formerly EHLR
IEP = Individualized education program
OCR = Office of Civil Rights
OSEP = Office of Special Education Programs
OSERS = Office of Special Education and Rehabilitative Services
OT = Occupational therapy
Pub = Public
PDD = Pervasive developmental disorder
PT = Physical therapy
RA = Rheumatoid arthritis
Remanded = Higher court sends the case back to the trial court for further consideration or review
S Ct = Supreme Court
Sch = School
SEA = State Education Agency
Unilaterally = Action that occurred without the consent of the other party

Table 3. Court Decisions, Letters of Inquiry, and Policy Interpretation Related to School-Based Physical Therapy: Federal District Court Decisions

Case	Citation	Jurisdiction/Year	Issue	Comments
John M. by Christine M. and Michael M. v. Board of Educ. of Evanston Community Consolidated Sch. Dist. 65	37 IDELR 38	N.D IL 2002	Reimbursement for PT	PT goals were found to be vague, but student received services 60 minutes/week. Court awarded family reimbursement for independent education evaluations, including one for PT.
Gulbrandsen by Gulbrandsen v. Conejo Valley Unified Sch.	36 IDELR 126	C.D. CA 2001	Adequacy of PT services	School district ordered to provide PT services once a week for 60 minutes for remainder of school year because of district's failure to provide FAPE and improperly challenging the PT assessment findings.
Moubry v. Independent Sch. Dist. No. 696	33 IDELR 92	D. Minn 2000	Reduction of PT services	School district evaluations to document student progress and needs were appropriate, as was district's reduction of PT services. School district had appropriately notified parents of service reductions, but reinstated prior level of services when parents requested due process.
TR vs Kingwood Township Board of Education	30 IDELR 1	DNJ 1999	Location of PT services	School was not required to provide PT at the private school because it would cost more to provide therapy at the private school than at the public school.
River Forest Sch. Dist. No. 90 v Illinois State Bd. of Education	24 IDELR 36	N.D. Ill. 1996	Medical versus educational PT services & reimbursement for PT services	Physical therapy provided at two rehabilitation facilities was determined to have an educational component and "just because that therapy was not provided in a classical academic environment did not render it medical in nature." In addition, the court determined that the parents could not be required to use their personal insurance if it would result in a threat of financial loss; however, the court did not have enough information to determine if such a financial loss would occur, so a trial on that specific issue would be required.
Crider v Bayard City Sch.	553 N.W.2d 147	D. Neb. 1996	Adequacy of PT services	Parents were required to exhaust administrative remedies before proceeding with negligence claim related to provision of contracted PT services.
Kerry B. v Union 53 Pub. Sch.	882 F. Supp. 184	D. Mass. 1995	Compensatory PT services	Student awarded compensatory PT services when the hearing revealed that PT did not commence in a timely fashion.
Howell v Waterford Pub. Schs.	731 F. Supp. 1314	E.D. Mich. 1990	Adequacy of PT services	Requirement to exhaust administrative remedies prior to pursuing civil action had not been met.
Holmes v Sobol	690 F. Supp. 154	W.D.N.Y. 1988	Extended school year services	PT was required during summer months when absence of therapy would delay progress towards IEP goals.
Maurits v Board of Educ. of Harford County	1983-1984 EHLR, DEC. 555:364	D. Md. 1983	PT not a required related service	A student with hemophilia was not entitled to special education and related services, because his illness did not affect his academic performance. Therefore, he did not qualify for school-based PT.

Table 4. Court Decisions, Letters of Inquiry, and Policy Interpretation Related to School-Based Physical Therapy: State Courts Decisions

Case	Citation	Jurisdiction/Year	Issue	Comments
Central Bucks Sch. Dist v Sara K by Mr and Mrs K	34 IDELR 235	Pa. Commonw. Ct, 2000	Compensatory education and PT services	School district's failure to provide 7-year-old student with PDD and autism with the appropriate number of PT sessions and ESY services resulted in student regression and justified compensatory services.
Giventer by Giventer V v Rementeria	32 IDELR 65	NY S Ct., 2000	Compensation for PT services	Therapy service provided to a student with severe brain damage under IDEA would not reduce the medical malpractice damages awarded to the student for services outside the school-based setting.
Crider by Crider v Bayard City Sch	24 IDELR 948	NE S Ct, 1996	Adequacy and discontinuation of PT	Parents did not show valid cause of action when alleging that 3 public agencies were negligent in failing to provide PT services to a student with multiple disabilities, but the court granted the parents permission to amend their complaint to correct their deficiencies.
Pittsburgh Bd. of Educ v Commonwealth Dep't of Educ	581 A 2d 681	Pa Commonw Ct, 1990	Compensatory PT services	Compensatory services were awarded after the school district unilaterally discontinued therapy services.

Table 5. Court Decisions, Letters of Inquiry, and Policy Interpretation Related to School-Based Physical Therapy: State Education Agencies (SEA) Decisions

Case	Citation	Jurisdiction/Year	Issue	Comments
Somerset County Pub. Schs.	48 IDELR 27	SEA MD 2007	Compensatory PT services	District had to provide compensatory PT services when they did not implement PT services for a 17-year-old student with CP for the first 3 months of the school year, despite their reasonable efforts to hire a part-time PT. District was also asked to consider compensatory education services for missed instructional time traveling to neighboring county to receive PT services.
Glendor Unified Sch. Dist.	46 IDELR 300	SEA CA 2006	Termination of PT services	District did not take "student's unique educational needs into account before terminating PT services for a 6-year-old student. District did not show that PT (and OT) services assisted student to overcome identified limitations.
Ysleta Indep. Sch. Dist.	43 IDELR 19	SEA TX 2004	Adequacy of PT services	District appropriately provided PT, as well as other related services, through consultation by showing "meaningful benefit." Student's slow progress was contributed to the severity of his multiple disabilities, not inappropriate related services.
Corpus Christi Indep. Sch. Dist.	4 ECLPR 452	SEA TX 2003	Termination of PT services	School district ordered to continue aqua therapy that had been previously provided by PT and OT over the past two years. District's attempts to separate aqua therapy from land-based PT and OT was determined inappropriate.
Alexandria Community Sch. Corp.	4 ECLPR 441	SEA IN 2003	Adequacy of PT services	Parents request to increase services to two times per week was denied, as was their request for ESY PT services because child was developing gross motor skills with current levels of service and no indication of regression over the summer existed.
Capistrano Unified Sch. Dist.	4 ECLPR 438	SEA CA 2003	PT evaluation timelines	Plan for PT services was not completed before meeting, resulting in denial of FAPE.
West Memphis Sch. Dist.	38 IDELR 222	SEA AR 2003	Compensatory PT services	District did not provide PT as indicated in IEP, including failure to initiate services until several months of school year had passed. School ordered to develop plan for providing compensatory PT services.
Greene County Bd. of Educ.	4 ECLPR 418	SEA AL 2002	Adequacy of PT services and compensatory PT	Child awarded compensatory services, including PT and district ordered to "redraft the IEP" because IEP did not contain specific information re: PT and other services and did not specify "who, where, when, and how" services would be provided.
Brown Deer Sch. Dist.	36 IDELR 176	SEA WI 2001	Adequacy of staff qualifications, physical facilities and equipment	Parents alleged that district denied FAPE when they failed to provide a safe learning environment after their child's leg was broken during school therapy session. The district requested dismissal of the allegations, but the judge ruled that relief may be granted under IDEA.
Fontana Unified Sch. Dist.	36 IDELR 78	SEA CA 2001	Adequacy of PT services	Related services, including PT, were adequately provided in the classroom and monitored by PT. PT services did not have to be provided after student's 21st birthday.
Georgetown County Sch. Dist.	4 ECLPR 344	SEA SC 2001	PT evaluation	District required to pay for PT and other evaluations to facilitate development of IEP and to determine how applied behavior analysis could be enhanced in educational program.

Table 5. Court Decisions, Letters of Inquiry, and Policy Interpretation Related to School-Based Physical Therapy: State Education Agencies (SEA) Decisions (continued)

Case	Citation	Jurisdiction/Year	Issue	Comments
Arlington Indep. Sch. Dist.	35 IDELR 298	SEA TX 2001	Adequacy of PT services	Parent was unable to show that the school denied child PT services.
Hickory Pub. Schs.	35 IDELR 141	SEA NC 2001	Discontinuation of PT services	District sought to discontinue PT services, but parents showed that eliminating the services would prevent son from benefiting from special education and district's expert agreed that lack of PT services would cause mobility declines.
Board of Educ. of the Monroe-Woodbury Cent. Sch. Dist	4 ECLPR 325	SEA NY 2001	Adequacy of PT services and compensatory services	District ordered to review educational program and determine additional amounts of service for the student due to district's failure to provide the services, including PT, included on the child's IEP.
Elmhurst Pub Schs. Community Unit Dist. 205	35 IDELR 136	SEA IL 2001	Adequacy of PT services and compensatory services	District had to amend IEP to include conductive education for 3 hours/day because student did not make progress with district's therapy programs and IEP did not adequately measure progress. Parents were reimbursed for their costs of providing related services for two school years and two summers.
Board of Educ. of the Syosset Cent. Sch. Dist.	4 ECLPR 312	SEA NY 2001	IEP content	District had to reimburse parents for services they sought because district's IEP did not include goals and objectives for special education and related services, including PT. A second IEP developed by a board failed to address goals and objectives that PT would support.
Hatfield Pub. Schs.	34 IDELR 168	SEA MA 2001	Discontinuation of PT services	Parent sought to discontinue PT services for 12-year-old student; however, district was required to reevaluate the student to determine what, if any, regression had occurred and to address the "amount and nature" of PT that would be necessary to address regression.
Kirby Sch. Dist. #140	34 IDELR 82	SEA ILL 2000	Adequacy of PT services and IEP	District ordered to include conductive education as part of IEP because of the lack of progress in PT program for student with cerebral palsy. IEP was not "reasonably calculated to confer educational benefit" because of the district's failure to address PT and other related services.
Board of Educ. of the Weedsport Cent. Sch. Dist.	31 IDELR 125	SEA NY 1999	Adequacy of PT services and IEP goals	The IEP goals for physical therapy to address wheelchair mobility were found to be adequate for a 10-year-old student with athetoid cerebral palsy.
Limestone County Bd. of Educ.	31 IDELR 122	SEA AL 1999	Adequacy of PT services	PT services for a 7-year-old with multiple disabilities were appropriate with regard to both frequency and content, and the school district was not obligated to provide a full-time aide during the child's participation in her regular classroom.
Cent. Sch. Dist. School City of E. Chicago	31 IDELR 45	SEA IN 1998	Frequency of PT services	PT services were provided as required in 14 year old's IEP; however, services were not provided on the day or at the time on student's schedule and were not well documented. School was ordered to report the student's progress in attainment of goals to the guardian.
Montgomery County Public School	30 IDELR 287	SEA MD 1998	Frequency of PT services	Parents alleged that 30 min per week of PT was not sufficient for their 11-year-old student with multiple disabilities. The hearing officer concluded that the proposed amount of PT was insufficient and directed that the school provide 1 hour per week.

Table 5. Court Decisions, Letters of Inquiry, and Policy Interpretation Related to School-Based Physical Therapy: State Education Agencies (SEA) Decisions (continued)

Case	Citation	Jurisdiction/Year	Issue	Comments
Muscogee County School District	30 IDELR 75	SEA GA 1999	Adequacy and reimbursement of PT services	PT services provided to a high school student with spastic diplegic CP provided FAPE and parent request for district funded therapy outside the school was denied.
Siskiyou County Office of Educ.	29 IDELR 113	SEA CA 1998	Adequacy of PT services	School district and parents disagreed about the amount of PT services a 9-year-old student with developmental delays needed. The IEP included physical therapy for 2 hours per month. The hearing officer determined the proposed amount of physical therapy was adequate.
Tucson Unified Sch. Dist.	28 IDELR 116	SEA AZ 1998	Compensatory services & reimbursement	The hearing officer determined that a school had provided FAPE when OT services specified in an interim IEP were provided by a physical therapist because the PT was qualified and worked on the student's IEP goal and objectives. The hearing officer denied compensatory services and reimbursement for the costs of private school placement.
Watson Chapel Sch. Dist.	27 IDELR 899	SEA AR 1998	Compensatory services & extended year services	A school district was not required to provide compensatory therapy (PT and OT) services for a 7-year-old with mental retardation and ADHD because the parents prevented the district from completing evaluations and providing services in a timely manner. However, the school district had to provide compensatory services in the form of extended year services because it failed to do so in the previous year.
Board of Educ. of the Lynbrook Union Free Sch. Dist.	27 IDELR 98	SEA NY 1997	Provision of PT after school hours	A parent's request to provide PT services outside school hours was denied by the hearing officer, as provision of physical therapy during school hours did not deny a FAPE.
Board of Educ. of the Canastoga Cent. Sch. Dist.	27 IDELR 419	SEA NY 1997	Reduction of PT services	The IEP developed by a school district that reduced the amount of PT and OT provided was found to be appropriate.
Laredo Indep. Sch. Dist.	27 IDELR 856	SEA TX 1997	PT not a required related service	An 8-year-old student with CP and ADHD did not require OT, PT, or a laptop computer. Although the student had a slight impairment of his gross motor skills, it did not affect his ability to progress in the educational environment.
Dallas Sch. Dist.	27 IDELR 873	SEA PA 1997	Service providers	The district was allowed to make changes in a child's PT service provider as long as the new providers had appropriate certification and licenses. The change in PT service providers did not prevent the provision of a FAPE.
Conecuh County Sch. Bd.	27 IDELR 112	SEA AL 1997	Adequacy of services	A school district failed to provide an 11-year-old student with mental retardation, speech impairment, and other health impairment with adequate related services. The school district had been provided several recommendations for the provision OT and PT, the district failed to address the need for such services. OT services provided in an "indirect manner" were found insufficient. PT services were not required based on two evaluations, but district was required to review the student's needs at the end of the school year.

Table 5. Court Decisions, Letters of Inquiry, and Policy Interpretation Related to School-Based Physical Therapy: State Education Agencies (SEA) Decisions (continued)

Case	Citation	Jurisdiction/Year	Issue	Comments
Corpus Christi Indep. Sch. Dist.	26 IDELR 658	SEA TX 1997	Extended year services & adequacy of PT services	Hearing officer determined that 30 minutes of PT every 6 weeks was insufficient for an 8-year-old student with mental retardation, an orthopedic impairment, a speech impairment, and other health impairment. The school was required to provide additional PT. The district was also required to provide extended year services, as the student would experience significant regression without such services.
Duneland Sch. Corp.	26 IDELR 1211	SEA IN 1997	Adequacy of PT services	The school district's proposed 30-45 minutes of PT per week were insufficient for a 10-year-old with CP and a learning disability. The school district was required to provide 3 sessions of PT per week and 1 session per week during the summer.
Los Angeles Unified Sch. Dist.	26 IDELR 618	SEA CA 1997	Discontinuation of PT services	The school district appropriately discontinued PT services for an 8-year-old student with a traumatic brain injury based on the results of the district PT, two physicians, and an outside PT evaluation.
Mount Horeb Area Sch.Dist.	25 IDELR 286	SEA WI 1997	Discontinuation of PT services	The school district appropriately discontinued PT services for a 7th grade student with emotional disturbance, as "neither 'postural slouching' nor illegible handwriting gave rise to the need for OT/PT."
Dallas Indep. Sch. Dist.	25 IDELR 1021	SEA TX 1997	Adequacy of PT services	The district was not required to have a licensed physical therapist provide range of motion for a student with multiple disabilities, mental retardation, and a visual impairment. The physical therapy program provided by the district was appropriate, including both direct and consultative services.
Board of Educ. Of the Enlarged City Sch. Dist. of the City of Cortland	24 IDELR 787	SEA NY 1996	Third-party reimbursement	School district did not have to reimburse an insurance company for its expenditures for related services.
West Milford Bd. of Educ.	24 IDELR 608	SEA NJ 1996	Adequacy of PT services	Parent was not entitled to reimbursement for PT services obtained privately because the parent interfered by terminating the child's in-school therapy after the board refused to allow the parent to observe sessions without an appointment. Any videotaping of sessions was to be done by the school—not the parents.
Muscogee County Sch. Dist.	22 IDELR 204	SEA GA 1995	Adequacy of PT services	District's efforts to make up PT services not provided in the previous school year due to staffing problems were found to be adequate and did not deny FAPE.
Brookings Sch. Dist.	22 IDELR 1099	SEA SD 1995	Compensatory services	District failed to provide interim therapy coverage while attempting to fill a personnel vacancy.
East Windsor Bd. of Educ.	20 IDELR 1478	SEA CT 1994	Type of PT service	Benefits derived from horseback riding could be adequately addressed in the school district's (more traditional) PT program.
In re Child with Disabilities	21 IDELR 594	SEA CT 1994	Adequacy of PT services and compensatory services	School district required to provide additional PT and to reimburse parents for supplementing the student's program after reducing PT services for administrative expediency.
Westminster Sch. Dist.	21 IDELR 398	SEA CA 1994	Adequacy of PT services	Student with severe disabilities entitled to PT services and an augmentative communication specialist.

Table 5. Court Decisions, Letters of Inquiry, and Policy Interpretation Related to School-Based Physical Therapy: State Education Agencies (SEA) Decisions (continued)

Case	Citation	Jurisdiction/Year	Issue	Comments
Huntsville City Bd. of Educ.	18 IDELR 1243	SEA AL 1992	Need for intensive therapy services	Parental request for residential placement for intensive therapy services was not calculated to provide educational benefit.
Hayward Unified Sch. Dist.	16 EHLR 277	SEA CA. 1989	Service provider	OT required to develop an appropriate feeding program, and PT could be trained to implement the program. Use of only a PT who was trained in feeding was not acceptable.
Rochester City Bd. of Educ.	1987-1988 EHLR DEC. 509:268	SEA NY 1988	Extended school year services	Summer PT was not required because it would only treat the physiological condition and would not enhance the educational program.
Grand Prairie Indep. Sch. Dist.	1986-1987 EHLR DEC. 508:317	SEA TX 1987	Qualifications and training of service providers	School district violated state law by permitting a homebound instructor to provide physical therapy services.
Fullerton Elementary Sch. Dist.	1986-1987 EHLR DEC. 508:255	SEA CA. 1986	Consultative services appropriate	Consultative services for preschooler with Down syndrome met the requirement of providing educational benefit. Reimbursement for direct services was denied.
Escambia County Sch. Bd.	1984-1985 EHLR DEC. 506:362	SEA FL. 1985	Assigned placement	School district may require all students who need PT to attend a particular school, so long as opportunities for being educated with nondisabled peers exist.
Los Angeles Unified Sch. Dist.	1985-1986 EHLR DEC. 507:117	SEA CA. 1985	Adequacy of PT services	Student with severe mental retardation required PT services.
Vallejo City Unified Sch. Dist.	1985-1986 EHLR DEC. 507:197	SEA CA. 1985	Consultative PT services were not appropriate	Direct intervention was required to meet the child's needs.
In re Child with Disability	1985-1986 EHLR DEC. 507:115	SEA IL 1985	Service provider	Physician's recommendation of a particular therapist was upheld when district did not conduct an evaluation to show that a change of therapist would not be harmful.
In re Child with Disability	1985-1986 EHLR DEC. 507:171	SEA IL 1985	Extended school year services	PT services required during the summer when required for educational and medical reasons.

Table 6. Court Decisions, Letters of Inquiry, and Policy Interpretation Related to School-Based Physical Therapy: Federal Agencies (OSEP, OSERS, OCR)

Case	Citation	Jurisdiction/Year	Issue	Comments
Letter to Geigerman	43 IDELR 85	OSEP 2004	PT as a related service	OSEP clarified that PT was a related service and that determination of whether PT is required is made by IEP team on a case-by-case basis and not based solely on the child's disability. Further clarified if services are required, then they must be included in IEP. Also explained that IEP teams are not required to comply with parental requests for services unless team determines related services are necessary for FAPE and that parents who disagree with IEP team decision have a right to due process.
Letter to Gully	42 IDELR 38	OSEP 2004	PT as an early intervention service	PT provided under Part C "is limited to those that are necessary to enable the child to benefit from other early intervention services." A child who has a major operation may require reevaluation to determine need for service changes and the IFSP team should meet to determine whether a change in services is required and whether such services are "purely medical in nature." If a change is required to support child's developmental and functional skills and not just a temporary need to recover from surgery, then those services would most likely be considered early intervention services.
Lake Ray Hubbard (TS) Shared	39 IDELR 74	OCR 2003	Compensatory PT services	District voluntarily agreed to provide middle school student with CP 13 hours of compensatory PT services because services did not start at the beginning of the school year due to a therapist's resignation. District found to have violated Section 504 and Americans with Disabilities Act by limiting student's access to school stage, water fountains, restrooms, walkway, and accessible parking spaces and agreed to make necessary changes.
Letter to Dickman	37 IDELR 284	OSEP 2002	Qualifications of providers	OSEP clarified that parents do not have a specific right under IDEA to be provided with the qualifications of the personnel providing services, but that the IEP team can include specific training, expertise and/or knowledge in a child's IEP, if necessary for the child to receive FAPE. Parents can request information regarding professional and/or paraprofessional qualifications of their child's classroom teacher and/or paraprofessional, under the No Child Left Behind Act.
Salem (MA) Pub. Schs.	37 IDELR 192	OCR 2002	Adequacy of PT room and equipment	Parent believed PT room was too small and district failed to provide adequate PT equipment to meet her son's needs. OCR determined that district provided adequate space and equipment to deliver individualize services to students. School district agreed to purchase a new floor exercise mat to assist in meeting PT goals contained on IEP.
Ketchikan (AK) Gateway Borough	35 IDELR 67	OCR 2001	PT evaluation and timelines	The district agreed to schedule a PT assessment and meet regarding results within 2 weeks of receipt to determine what additional supports the student may require.
Walton County (FL) Sch. Dist.	32 IDELR 262	OCR 2000	Compensatory education and PT evaluation	The district agreed to evaluate student's need for compensatory education and physical therapy and to provide such services if necessary.

Table 6. Court Decisions, Letters of Inquiry, and Policy Interpretation Related to School-Based Physical Therapy: Federal Agencies (OSEP,OSERS, OCR) (continued)

Case	Citation	Jurisdiction/Year	Issue	Comments
Puerto Rico (PR) Dept. of Education	31 IDELR 194	OCR 1999	Educational evaluation	Parents alleged that the school failed to complete a special education evaluation. As part of a resolution, the district agreed to continue to provide PT along with other services in the IEP and awarded compensatory service for the 8-month period when child did not receive PT.
St. Tammany (LA) Parish Sch. Bd.	31 IDELR 144	OCR 1999	Discrimination	Parents alleged discrimination because school district would not pay for related service provided by private therapists to a student with multiple disabilities, but did not present sufficient evidence to support their claim.
Lowndes County (AL) Sch. Dist	29 IDELR 485	OCR 1998	Provision of PT services	School district allegedly did not provide PT services unless they received an independent evaluation to identify the need for therapy. The school district entered into a resolution agreement to resolve the PT service issue.
Dade Count (FL) Sch. Dist.	27 IDELR 223	OCR 1997	Reduction of PT services	A school district's reduction in PT services was not discrimination. The parent's refusal to provide access to the residence interfered with the district's ability to provide appropriate services.
Weslaco (TX) Indep. Sch. Dist.	26 IDELR 1307	OCR 1997	Provision of PT services	A school district's decision not to provide physical therapy was not reviewed, as the district had provided the parent with information regarding the right to request an impartial hearing about the district's determination, including the procedures by which the parent could challenge the decision.
Rockdale County (GA) Sch. Dist.	22 IDELR 1047	OCR 1995	Discrimination	Parental request to discontinue PT and adaptive physical education was met, but these provisions were not removed from the IEP.
Letter to Graham	22 IDELR 502	OSEP 1994	Provision of PT services	Children unilaterally placed in private schools are to be afforded "a genuine opportunity for equitable participation." PT is a related service under Part B IDEA, but it may be defined as special education and necessary for FAPE under a state's own laws.
Capistrano (CA) Unified Sch. Dist.	21 IDELR 807	OCR 1994	Adequacy of PT services	Failure to specify the amount of services on the IEP and to provide these services was a violation of Section 504. Even though the school district attempted to meet its obligation for therapy services through a contractual arrangement with therapists, the district continues to be responsible for ensuring the appropriate amount of service is actually provided.
Norwalk (CT) Bd. of Educ.	21 IDELR 853	OCR 1994	Adequacy of PT services	Failure to provide direct intervention during the first week of school was satisfied by the therapist's attendance at other meetings directly related to the student's needs.
Summers County (WV) Sch.	20 IDELR 1362	OCR 1993	Consultative PT services appropriate	Consultative services were adequate to meet the student's needs unless there would be a change in condition.

Table 6. Court Decisions, Letters of Inquiry, and Policy Interpretation Related to School-Based Physical Therapy: Federal Agencies (OSEP,OSERS, OCR) (continued)

Case	Citation	Jurisdiction/Year	Issue	Comments
Letter from Rainforth	17 EHLR 222	OSEP 1990	Provision of related services or determination of need for related services	Schrag responded that "any guideline or other policy which, as written or implemented, acts as a categorical denial of related services to all students whose language or motoric skills are as delayed as their general developmental level, would be inconsistent with the requirements of the EHA-B. Such a categorical limitation on services would conflict with the EHA-B requirement that the services to be included in each student's IEP be determined on an individual basis."
Mineral County (WV) Sch.	16 EHLR 904	OCR 1990	Adequacy of PT services	School district failed to document or provide adequate services or to make placement decisions with the input from a group of knowledgeable persons.
Letter to Anonymous	EHLR 213:273	OSERS 1989	PT working conditions	Caseloads, frequency of services, use of aides, and place of provision are not addressed in EHA (prior to IDEA). State law may provide additional clarification on some of these matters.
Ripley-Ohio-Dearborn (IN) Special Educ. Cooperative	EHLR 353:281	OCR 1989	Need for service assessed by educational agency	Cooperative found to be in violation for lack of arranging, directing, and providing assessments for PT and OT.
Linden (CA) Unified Sch. Dist.	EHLR 352:617	OCR 1988	Policy on evaluation	District's policy not to evaluate students who were not disabled was a violation. Student with juvenile R.A. who did not qualify for special education was entitled to an evaluation.
Richmond (CA) Unified Sch. Dist.	EHLR 352:619	OCR 1988	FAPE denied	District did not provide replacement therapy or notify parents of discontinued services or transportation to alternative therapy site.
San Francisco (CA) Unified Sch. Dist.	EHLR 352:611	OCR 1988	Adequacy of PT services	Six-week interruption in therapy was not a violation since attempts had been made to find a replacement.
Letter to Butler	EHLR 213:118	OSERS 1988	PT required as a related service	Both PT and OT are required as related services to assist a child with disabilities to benefit from special education.
Eastern Upper Peninsula (MI) Intermediate Sch. Dist.	EHLR 352:538	OCR 1987	Adequacy of PT services	Failure to provide PT for 2 years was not justified by district's inability to hire or keep a qualified therapist.
Sumner County (TN) Sch. Dist.	EHLR 352:248	OCR 1986	Service provider	Services provided by a teacher and aide under the direction of a licensed PT and in conformity with state regulations was not in violation.